P9-CDS-167

AFTER *the*
ERROR

AFTER *the* ERROR

SPEAKING OUT
about patient safety
TO SAVE LIVES

Susan McIver, PhD *&*
Robin Wyndham

DISCARD

ECW Press

Copyright © Susan McIver and Robin Wyndham, 2013

Published by ECW Press
2120 Queen Street East, Suite 200, Toronto, Ontario, Canada M4E 1E2
416-694-3348 / info@ecwpress.com

All rights reserved. No part of this publication may be reproduced, stored in a retrieval system, or transmitted in any form by any process — electronic, mechanical, photocopying, recording, or otherwise — without the prior written permission of the copyright owners and ECW Press. The scanning, uploading, and distribution of this book via the Internet or via any other means without the permission of the publisher is illegal and punishable by law. Please purchase only authorized electronic editions, and do not participate in or encourage electronic piracy of copyrighted materials. Your support of the author's rights is appreciated.

LIBRARY AND ARCHIVES CANADA CATALOGUING IN PUBLICATION

McIver, Susan B. (Susan Bertha), 1940–
After the error : speaking out about patient safety to save
lives / Susan McIver.

Includes bibliographical references.
ISBN 978-1-77041-110-4
ALSO ISSUED AS: 978-1-77090-357-9 (PDF); 978-1-77090-358-6 (EPUB)

1. Medical errors—Canada. 2. Medical errors—Canada—
Prevention. 3. Patients—Safety measures. I. Title.

R729.8.M24 2013   362.10971   C2012-907526-4

Cover image: stefanolunardi/Shutterstock
Text design: Tania Craan
Cover design and production: Carolyn McNeillie
Printing: Friesens   5   4   3   2

ECW Press acknowledges the financial support of the Government of Canada through the Canada Book Fund for our publishing activities, and the contribution of the Government of Ontario through the Ontario Book Publishing Tax Credit. The marketing of this book was made possible with the support of the Ontario Media Development Corporation.

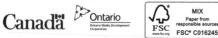

PRINTED AND BOUND IN CANADA

For Georgina Hunter

Her personal courage helped usher in a new era in the awareness of medical errors and showed that even one person has the power to create significant change.

"When you speak the unspeakable, something is lost and something is gained. I lost years of my life, but I gained a priceless connection with ethical, caring people." — Georgina Hunter

ACKNOWLEDGEMENTS

We would like to thank the contributors to this book, who were willing to share both their pain and their accomplishments and to persevere through the lengthy writing and editing process. Each one, in a unique way, helped to demonstrate that although medical errors do occur, it is possible to step outside of one's grief, anger and comfort zone to provide education to the public as well as work for changes in systems, laws and attitudes.

Many friends, relatives and associates have encouraged us in a variety of ways. We would like to mention and thank Georgina Hunter, Harry Goldhar and Dorothy Harp.

Helen Haskell assisted us by contacting potential contributors and providing support during this project.

We would like to especially acknowledge and thank Rhonda Nixon for the role she has played in generously assisting and supporting us over the past three years. Her experience, efforts and friendship were essential to the concept and preparation of this book.

We are indebted to Jack David for seeing the potential in our original concept and accepting this work for publication. The manuscript was greatly improved by the editorial assistance of Crissy Boylan and Kathleen Fraser. Erin Creasey and Athmika Punja deserve mention for their diligence and professionalism in promotion, sales and marketing. Thanks also to Carolyn McNeillie for the cover graphics and Sarah Dunn for publicity.

CONTENTS

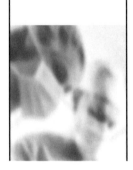

DISCLAIMER

This book contains stories documenting contributors' experiences with medical professionals. The authors have taken reasonable steps to verify the contributors' accounts, and each contributor has declared that the stories are true and accurate. Readers are advised not to rely in any way on the specific facts portrayed in any of the accounts and are prohibited from reproducing, publishing, translating and in any way commercially dealing with, in any medium, the accounts or any portion thereof without the written permission of the authors and the publisher.

A few of the stories in this book were written by the contributors; most were prepared by the authors based on personal interviews, telephone conversations, emails, newspaper and magazine articles, coroners' reports, medical records, books and articles, notes and rough drafts.

When a plane crashes, it is national, if not international, news. The question invariably posed is "How did this happen?" The television reporter, standing near the site of the crash, tells us that the black box is being located and that its contents will be meticulously examined for clues about what went wrong.

A 2012 study estimated that 40,000 Canadian patients die every year as a result of medical error. That is the equivalent of 80 jumbo jets crashing every year — one every five days or so. If a plane was crashing every five days, would anybody ever fly? Yet while individual cases of medical error do make headlines, the sheer and unacceptable scale of this worldwide problem is something that most people simply cannot comprehend.

Each story in this book is a black box. Each is a tragedy. But each is also a treasure trove, offering clues about what went wrong. You need only read two or three stories before patterns start to emerge. This book offers lessons, not just about what went wrong in each of these cases, but also about what is going wrong across the world's health-care systems, and about the factors that transpire to cause tragedy in the very places where we seek relief when we are sick.

A plane's black box records every bit of data imaginable about the flight in real time. It also records the voices of those at the centre of the unfolding tragedy — the pilots in the cockpit. This book tells the stories of those at the centre of their own unfolding tragedies. In most of the cases, these people died. This book gives them a voice.

When I founded the World Health Organization's first ever program on patient safety, it was the stories of patients and their relatives that motivated me. I vividly recollect even small details of their descriptions. This book exists because people have volunteered to share their most painful experiences. In doing so, they offer up a challenge to the health-care community, which is to eke out every possible piece of learning from these stories, so that they do not just remain as tragic stories but provide the basis on which improvements are made.

At the centre of this book is the difficult truth that thousands of people die unnecessarily in the hands of our health-care systems. Sometimes these are people who were critically unwell, but often they are people who were not. Yet interwoven through this book are also stories of hope and of individuals who have used their own experiences as a force for good, who have shared their stories so that others may avoid the same fate. The title of this book attests to its ambition — to speak out about patient safety, so that lives may be saved. As you read this book, please think hard. Think what went wrong. Think what needs to change. If we can collectively do this, and act on what we learn, we can make our health-care systems as safe as our airlines are.

Professor Sir Liam Donaldson
World Health Organization
Envoy for Patient Safety

It takes courage to speak out about medical errors. It takes persistence, stamina and support from others to effect change. This book was written to recognize the patients and families whose activities have helped to lay the foundation of current patient safety programs and who continue to raise awareness, identify problems and provide solutions. Their accomplishments have often come at considerable emotional, psychological and financial expense. Their stories provide examples of what can be done to promote safer health care and also remind readers that in spite of increasing efforts to prevent errors, they continue to devastate lives. The contributors are all Canadians; however, their experiences and achievements speak to the world.

American patients and media have played a significant role in drawing attention to medical errors. In the 1970s and 1980s, medical malpractice claims associated with anesthesia accounted for a disproportionately high payout of medical liability insurance. In the early 1980s, national media publicity turned a harsh spotlight on injuries associated with anesthesia. The Anesthesia Patient Safety Foundation (APSF) was established in 1985 to address these concerns and as a result anesthesiologists have become widely recognized as pioneering leaders in patient safety.

In 1999, the Institute of Medicine (IOM) of the U.S. National Academy of Sciences released its landmark report, *To Err Is Human: Building a Safer Health Care System*.[1] The report stated that 44,000 to 98,000 preventable deaths occur annually because of medical errors in hospitals alone. At the time, these numbers were startling; however, more recent studies have found medical errors to be much more prevalent.

A survey completed in 2012 revealed that almost one third of Americans reported that either they or a friend or family member had experienced a medical error.[2] Based on a population of approximately 320 million, this survey indicated that close to 100 million Americans have had direct or indirect experience with medical errors. As many as 25 percent of all hospital patients are harmed by medical errors, according to a 2010 report.[3] The study found little evidence that efforts to reduce errors have translated into significant improvements in the overall safety of patients. In 2011, it was reported that adverse events occur in one third of hospital admissions.[4]

A Canadian study estimated that 7.5 percent of patients admitted to acute care hospitals in 2000 experienced one or more adverse events[5] and approximately 24,000 patients die annually as a result of adverse events that occur in hospitals. A 2009 report revealed that approximately one in six Canadians said they had experienced at least one error in the previous two years.[6] This translated to 4.2 million adult Canadians. Not all of these reported errors caused even minor harm, but their numbers clearly illustrate the magnitude of the problem.

A 2012 report stated that approximately 38,000 to 43,000 deaths occur annually in Canada in connection with health-care delivery.[7] According to the same report, the actual total number of deaths is undoubtedly much greater because of the high rates of non-reporting. In addition to those who die, there are hundreds of thousands of Canadians who are harmed from health-care delivery.

An Australian study reported in 1995 that there were approximately 230,000 preventable adverse events in hospitals each year, and as a result between 10,000 and 14,000 people died.[8] In 2000, a British study reported that adverse events harmed approximately 10 percent of patients admitted to hospital, or more than 850,000 individuals each year.[9] Many other countries have undertaken similar studies.

The financial costs of medical errors are inextricably intertwined with human suffering. In 2002, following a book reading that I (S.M.) gave in Kelowna, BC, I spoke to a distraught woman whose husband, a tradesman, had undergone what was supposed to be straightforward surgery on his elbow several years before. The surgeon nicked a blood vessel during surgery which eventually resulted in extensive tissue damage. In the intervening years, her husband was unable to work and had undergone another 23 surgeries, most involving sequential amputations of his fingers and eventually parts of his arm. The woman wept as she spoke of the emotional and financial impacts on her family. The wider impact was the cost of additional surgeries and related care, the loss of tax revenue and the loss of a skilled tradesman in the workforce.

A study on the economics of patient safety in acute care released in 2012 by the Canadian Patient Safety Institute (CPSI) estimated that the economic burden of preventable incidents for 2009–2010 was $397 million.[10] This estimate represented only a small portion of the entire cost of harmful incidents in Canada because it did not include the indirect costs of care after hospital discharge, or societal costs of illness such as loss of functional status or occupational productivity. Preventable medical errors may cost the United States up to $1 trillion dollars in lost human potential and contributions, according to a 2012 report.[11] Previous estimates of the annual cost of medical errors in the United States were in the tens of billions of dollars and focused on direct medical costs, including ancillary services, prescription drug services and inpatient and outpatient care.[11, 12]

Patient safety organizations dedicated to reporting, education, funding, advocacy and data collection have been established in a number of countries. (See For Further Information at page 250.) These organizations include those established by governments, private groups and individuals. In 2004, the World Health Organization launched the World Alliance for Patient Safety. Subsequently, Patients for Patient Safety was formed under the auspices of the World Alliance in order to involve patients as partners in improving safety in all health-care settings throughout the world. In Canada, Patients for Patient Safety is a program within the CPSI.

An increasing awareness of and concern about medical errors in Canada and globally is driving extensive efforts to understand why and how errors occur and how to prevent them. In this country, national and international conferences and symposia bring together experts to share their ideas. Graduate programs are being established and continuing education courses in patient safety at all levels help to train leaders in the field. Hospitals, health regions and professional associations all initiate and support programs in patient safety.

When patients enter the medical system, they expect that their illnesses will be cured, their broken bones will be mended and, if at the end of their lives, that they will die free of pain and at peace. They do not expect to experience infections, surgical mistakes or other complications in respected institutions staffed by people they trust to help them.

The chapters that follow in Part I provide true stories that are examples of various types of errors, their impact at a personal level and the efforts made to discover the truth in order to avoid further needless suffering. The chapters in Part II offer information on how to prevent errors when making end-of-life decisions, how to use the media and how to organize large amounts of information, such as medical records, in order to facilitate investigations. The final chapter offers insights into medical malpractice.

PART I

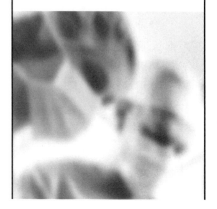

A Child Like Annie

Annie Farlow's 80-day-long life affected her parents and siblings in ways they never could have imagined. Her family, who had no previous experience with disabled children, loved Annie with all their hearts. When she died in August 2005, their grief was compounded by the discovery of circumstances associated with her care, which shattered their faith in her doctors and their hope that Annie would be seen as a person and not just as a syndrome. The Farlow family's experience answers the question that is so often asked of parents, both before and after a birth associated with genetically different children: Who wants a child like that anyway?

Annie's brief life transformed her mother Barbara into an internationally respected parental voice in pediatric ethics. Through Barbara's work, Annie's story led to the largest survey ever of parents who have children with similar disabilities and the inclusion of those findings in the medical literature, which was previously lacking the parental perspective.

Barbara has consistently encouraged a much-needed and important discussion about the issues of medical care provided to, or withheld from, infants born with genetic differences, both in hospital and in the broader medical community. She recognizes and respects that some parents might make different choices than she did when they learn that their unborn baby will have disabilities. Families may also differ in their attitudes toward *withholding treatment. Either way, their wishes should be respected through a process that is transparent and accountable.*

Barbara joined with leading health-care professionals, patient advocates, ethicists and policy makers to tackle questions made especially difficult in this time of increasing resource scarcity in health care. When is it appropriate to limit or withdraw potentially beneficial treatment? Who should make those decisions? How should decisions be made?

The Farlows wanted Annie to be provided with the same treatments and interventions as any child without a genetic label or disability would be offered. They believe doctors made unilateral decisions which should have been made openly and in consultation with them. As a result of the secrecy in which decisions seem to have been made, Annie may have been denied not only an opportunity for a longer life, but also timely palliative care.

The author of numerous publications in prestigious medical journals and other respected health-care publications, Barbara has spoken to scores of hospital associations, medical schools, advocacy groups and ethics conferences. She has made presentations to the United Nations High Commission on Human Rights, the World Health Organization and Pan-American Health Organization. Barbara appeared before the Canadian Parliamentary Committee on Palliative and Compassionate Care, and her husband, Tim, spoke before the Ontario Provincial Parliament's standing committee on social justice.

Annie

In early 2005, Barbara and Tim Farlow were faced with a choice that would shape the rest of their lives. High school sweethearts, the Farlows had five children at home who excelled in school and sports. They were financially comfortable, enjoyed excellent health and were delighted when they learned a new baby was on the way.

Prenatal screening at 21 weeks revealed that their baby girl had a condition called trisomy 13. Many children with this genetic condition die at or shortly after birth, primarily from brain and heart anomalies. Some, however, can live with varying levels of disability for years, even into adolescence.

The initial response from Barbara, who has degrees in engineering science and business administration, was to find a rational solution. Lacking any experience with disability, she and Tim began asking themselves tough questions. Would they be able to make the commitment to such a needy child? What about the impact on their other children? What if Annie died suddenly after only a few days, weeks or months? Would it all have been worth it?

Their thinking began to change as they investigated the world of families with trisomy children. They expected to find distraught, depressed parents exhausted from caring for children who merely existed and had no value to themselves or anyone else. They instead found that parents felt their lives were enriched by having such a child. Most of the disabled children were happy and progressing at their own pace. Siblings were spontaneously affectionate with and protective of their disabled brother or sister. Whether the parents had chosen not to terminate pregnancy or had received a diagnosis after birth, they all appeared to take great delight in their children. Upon the death of their disabled child, families were devastated.

The obstetrician asked Barbara why she would continue the pregnancy when she knew the baby was going to die. "I was unable to formulate a coherent response at the time," Barbara said several years later. "Now I can. From the moment I knew of my baby's existence, I loved her unconditionally. We would take her journey together, as a family. We named our daughter Annie."

The Farlows were fully aware that most parents in their situation would not have made the same choice. They also knew that doctors might not agree with their decision or understand it. Would Annie be seen as a baby requiring attention, and not as a syndrome, when needing medical care in the future? Would the doctors value her life as much as that of an able-bodied child? Barbara and Tim did not want treatment that would be burdensome or futile, and they did not want Annie to suffer. They did, however, want to ensure that treatment would not be withheld from Annie on the basis of her disability alone.

Seeking clarification, Barbara and Tim met with doctors from the cardiology, genetics and bioethics departments at the children's hospital before Annie's birth. They were assured that Annie would be treated like any other child. Treatment, including surgical intervention, would be given as required. The Farlows would be informed of risks and benefits and any decision would be theirs. They were told a policy was in place to deal with ethical conflicts should any arise. In fact, the policy that outlined the determination of levels of treatment and the process for resolving ethical dilemmas between families and doctors was described to them in detail. Later, after Annie's death, they would read what the bioethicist had written about them at that meeting: "Calm, articulate, logical, frames in *best interest logic*. Want to give baby every opportunity for quality of life . . . don't want life of suffering."

Annie was born at full term, May 25, 2005, weighing seven pounds, with Apgar scores of 8 and 9. Unlike many babies born with trisomy 13, Annie could see and hear and had normal strength. She breathed well on her own and did not have the common lethal brain and cardiac anomalies.

Late one night, while still basking in the recent news that Annie had a reasonably good prognosis, Tim chatted with a young doctor who had dropped by. The doctor wanted to know why Tim and Barbara wanted a disabled child to live. Tim had no patience with what the doctor was suggesting. "She's my daughter and we love her," he curtly replied. The topic was never brought up again.

Annie did have hypoglycemia, which kept her in hospital for her first six weeks. She was fed a high-calorie diet through a nasal gastric tube and given a small quantity of oxygen through nasal prongs. During this time, either Tim or Barbara was always with Annie. They had many opportunities to communicate with the medical and nursing staff and felt they had developed an excellent relationship with the primary pediatrician.

Barbara recalled an important meeting: "During our stay, there had been a team meeting. We expressed our wishes to consider whatever treatment Annie might need to prolong her life and nobody disagreed. We kept a large envelope with us at all times, filled with information and stories of other children like Annie just in case anyone needed to better understand our position. However, no issues arose and we had no reason not to believe that we were on the same page as all the clinicians."

Annie's siblings welcomed her home with a driveway full of encouraging chalk drawings and messages. "Annie kicks butt" was Barbara's favourite. With Annie at home, the family established a schedule so that someone was always with her. Tim took an indefinite leave from work. Eventually, the family adjusted to the new routine, Annie gained weight and at the age of 75 days she smiled for the first time.

The next day, Annie developed episodic respiratory distress and her face turned a permanent red. The Farlows immediately took her to the local senior regional pediatrician, who told them Annie's red face was a reaction to medication and the distress was caused by a floppy trachea. This pediatrician advised conservative management of the trachea, because the problem might resolve without treatment.

Annie's distress worsened the following day and the Farlows took her to the regional hospital, where the attending physician sent them to the children's hospital by ambulance. Barbara and Tim were relieved to find their primary-care pediatrician in the emergency room waiting for them. After the pediatrician and his team reviewed the results of blood work and x-rays, he said Annie had pneumonia. The Farlows considered this good news. Children can recover from pneumonia.

Several hours later, while on the ward, Annie suffered a respiratory crash. An arterial blood sample was taken and the Farlows were left alone with a therapist who manually ventilated Annie with a bag mask for over an hour before she was transferred to the pediatric intensive care unit (PICU).

Sixteen hours later, in the PICU, Annie's oxygen saturation numbers suddenly dropped. The therapist again manually ventilated her. The primary-care pediatrician and an intensivist arrived within minutes. The intensivist said the problem was *not* pneumonia. He told Tim and Barbara that Annie needed an operation, called a tracheoplasty, on her narrowed trachea. In this surgery, Annie's chest would be opened and cartilage from elsewhere in her body would be used to enlarge the trachea. The surgery had a very high mortality rate for children who did not have the challenges of a genetic condition like Annie's.

The intensivist asked them if he should intubate Annie. The Farlows turned to their trusted primary pediatrician for guidance. He advised against intubation for Annie. He stayed with the Farlows until Annie died a short time later at the age of 80 days. The same pediatrician spent time with Tim, Barbara and their children in the bereavement room.

Within days, Barbara's logical mind combined with her maternal instinct made her question the events in the emergency room. A team of highly qualified doctors had diagnosed pneumonia, yet 24 hours later the Farlows were told that the cause of Annie's respiratory distress was not pneumonia. "We had complete trust in Annie's doctors and they had been kind when she died. For these reasons, I felt guilty and ashamed to order the records as it seemed like an act of mistrust or disloyalty," Barbara said.

She took Annie's medical records to a friend who is a nurse practitioner. After examining the records, the nurse practitioner told them that hours before Annie's death, the intensivist had placed a do not resuscitate (DNR) order in Annie's records. This order had been placed without their knowledge or consent. In fact, the previous evening the Farlows had made it very clear to the same intensivist that they needed a diagnosis for Annie so they could make an informed decision and not live with regret. They told him that they had accepted Annie's predicted disabilities and that her life had value to their family.

The intensivist later provided his justification for placing the "do not resuscitate" order. In response to the parents' letter questioning the placement of the order without consent, he wrote, "a discussion with Mr. Farlow through the night and in the morning *suggested* that the parents' wishes *may be changing*" (authors' emphasis).

Barbara said:

> We had made our position clear; there was no ambiguity on the code status. During Annie's final admission, we were asked twice, "Is she DNR?" Each time we responded, "No! We need to know what is

wrong." The third time we were asked was in response to the same intensivist who eventually placed the DNR order without our consent. He asked if he should resuscitate if Annie stopped breathing. I said yes, because we had been told she had pneumonia, which most likely could be successfully treated. He then went on about "dying with dignity," but provided no information about Annie's condition. He asked for the DNR again. I told him that we were well aware of Annie's predicted disabilities and had accepted them. I told him her life had value to us. I said we didn't want her to live on machines, but we needed to know what was wrong and whether we could or should fix it. To our dismay and that of the nurse present, he stormed out of the room.

The nurse practitioner's examination of the records and subsequent investigations revealed additional issues. The diagnosis of pneumonia was not supported, as Annie's blood work did not show any infection. As well, the records stated that there was good air entry to both lungs and no consolidations (dense areas on x-rays) were observed. Several treatments less severe than the risky operation suggested by the intensivist were possible.

Annie had normal and stable vital signs minutes before her oxygen saturation levels plummeted in the PICU. Most of her final records, including her final medication record, were absent from the documents provided to Barbara.

Barbara later learned that Annie's carbon dioxide levels had been progressively critical commencing the fifth day after birth. A pulmonologist, concerned about Annie's trachea, had examined her at three weeks. He advised the pediatrician that two tests be done, a high KV x-ray and a fluoroscopy. The pediatrician did not order the first and cancelled his initial order for the second. As Barbara explained later, these tests would have ruled out the possibility that Annie's tracheal compression was caused by an artery. She was at risk for this, as noted in the records, because her heart was centred in her chest, giving rise to an increased probability of abnormal association of major arteries with the trachea.

The pulmonologist's advice and the pediatrician's decision not to follow it both occurred without the Farlows' knowledge. Doctors at two hospitals had apparently ignored the increasing carbon dioxide levels and said nothing to Barbara or Tim. Annie's red face was the result of these sustained critical levels. Annie had been heading for a respiratory crisis her entire life.

The official cause of Annie's death was given initially as "complications of trisomy 13." The new chief coroner, however, revised this and informed the Farlows by letter that the primary cause was "central hypoventilation." A private medical review referred to this condition as slow asphyxiation. The Farlows never learned the exact cause of Annie's final rapid decline or whether indeed she could still be sharing their lives. They had made the critical decision to let Annie die with the belief that she would not likely survive the surgery described, yet the coroner's report stated, "It was by no means certain she had to undergo prolonged burdensome interventions such as prolonged ventilation or distressful surgery."

Barbara recalled: "We were shocked and devastated and so hurt by the violation of trust in Annie's providers. We had trusted their competency and integrity without question. We learned years later that Annie's primary-care pediatrician had cared for a three-year-old with trisomy 13 just the summer before Annie's death. The family had fought a major battle just to have a specialist consult for a life-threatening condition. This child remains alive and well as of November 2011."

The Farlows kept hoping for an explanation, because what they were discovering could not possibly be true. But it was. They felt they had been deceived from the time of the meeting before Annie's birth, when they were assured she would be treated like any other child, through to the DNR decision being made without consulting them. In addition, their lack of involvement in the treatment plan ensured that Annie received neither appropriate life-saving care nor effective palliation. As Barbara said, these were award-winning physicians at a renowned children's hospital. She and Tim felt, however, that the physicians made a series of decisions during Annie's short life that reflected their belief that her life was not worth saving.

The coroner's pediatric death review committee did not support the Farlows' contention that necessary treatment was withheld from Annie and that a culture of withholding life-saving treatment for some infants is part of the hospital's culture. The committee did, however, state that "the events of the final 24 hours and the initiation of palliative care together with writing of a DNR order as stated above do not represent appropriate forms of care." The report also stated that "when the decision represents a major change in management, full documentation by caregivers is crucial. It was notably absent in this case."

The Farlows had one meeting with the doctors involved with Annie's care before the coroner's investigation began. After completion of the investigation, they made a request to meet with the doctors and offered to "sign anything" absolving the hospital of legal responsibility. With one notable exception, however, the doctors refused to meet with them. The senior pediatrician at the regional hospital continued communication with the family through emails. For that reason alone, the Farlows did not name her in the lawsuit they reluctantly brought against the hospital and doctors.

Regarding the lawsuit, Barbara said: "I think it is important to meet with the family until all questions have been answered. Apology, if necessary, should be made in person. This would be a much better solution than a lawsuit. The amount of the claim was $10,000. Children like Annie are worth very little in the legal system. The purpose of the lawsuit was to obtain accountability and remedies. It was a costly and altruistic endeavour."

A written apology from the hospital was eventually issued. Included was this statement: "Sometimes when we care for children such as Annie who have very complex care needs, communication does not occur in as clear and consistent fashion as we would wish. For that, we are very sorry."

In time, Barbara and Tim came to better understand the events that had occurred with Annie's medical care, including the failure to diagnose the cause of her serious ongoing respiratory condition and her slow death from asphyxiation.

Barbara reflected: "The situation likely was not as simple as making best-interest, informed medical decisions for Annie. There were other children and limited resources to consider, as well as value judgments and choices for her doctors to make. Hospital-based doctors have shared with me that there are economic pressures. When there is a bed shortage, it is like a macabre game of musical chairs. Who will get the last bed? How are these decisions made? In the system we encountered, it seemed to be the unanimous group think of the clinicians that Annie's life had no value. As economic pressures increase, as we know they will, what will become of children with lesser disabilities?"

Reflections and Achievements

Seven years after learning she was pregnant with a trisomy 13 baby, Barbara wrote:

> My husband and I could not be at peace to let Annie die without knowing if she had a chance to live a few happy years. We just needed a diagnosis, and if treatment was not in her best interest, we wanted her to have a dignified death. It really should not have been difficult. We made it clear that we did not want her to live on machines or suffer repeated intubations. I think we were easy parents to get along with.
>
> At the beginning, we truly believed that we would be able to resolve our concerns with the hospital. We just wanted them to establish a process whereby ethically challenging cases would be dealt with in a transparent manner resulting in either medical interventions or palliative care. I now understand that the issues are very complex and relate to politics, funding and values and these appear to conflict at times with public expectations and beliefs as set out by law and the UN Convention on the Rights of the Child.
>
> All along, we believed that we would reach the end of the journey in "the next month or so." Suddenly, it is six years later. What compelled me most to begin the journey were two comments made by Annie's doctors. A hospital vice-president told us that in one meeting about Annie, one of her doctors asked the others, "Who wants a child like that anyway?" Shortly after Annie died, we met with the senior

regional pediatrician. We told her that something very wrong seemed to have happened at the hospital. She sighed and said, "Sometimes a family just *doesn't get it*. I prefer not to deal with it so I send them to someone who can."

My pursuit continued because I continued to make more discoveries that I found alarming. An example is the government's Assistive Devices Program, which explicitly restricts infants who suffer from apnea as a result of a "pre-existing condition" from having an at-home apnea monitor.

In the fall, I attended a public bioethics talk at the hospital where Annie died about discharging, planning and community services. The speaker, who is a physician and policy strategist, explained to everyone how the government makes funding decisions and how the bottom line is that there will be no more money for community services for disabled children. She suggested that it was important to "think critically about quality of life versus salvageable life" and questioned whether 24-week preemies should be resuscitated. I was disturbed by this because I think these are societal decisions that need public and parental input.

One of the doctors I am working with was invited by the Academic Pediatric Societies to be on a panel on trisomy 18 at their annual meeting in Boston in spring 2012. She insisted that I also be on the panel to speak for the parents and they invited me. It was an incredible opportunity as it was a very influential conference.

This will hopefully complete the journey for me. I will have provided a voice for Annie and all of the children like her. I can't do more than that.

Annie's voice has helped to make improvements at the hospital level toward advance care-planning for children with complex needs. As Barbara said, however, the underlying problem of having to "choose" persists. In the broader medical community, she is concerned about the lack of input from parents when international guidelines are being established that recommend that children with disabilities like Annie's not be resuscitated at birth due to risk of an early death or unacceptably high morbidity.

Doctors have told Barbara that they rely almost exclusively on peer-reviewed medical literature for information. The literature is missing the parents' perceptions of the nature of their trisomy children and their experience of caring for them. A study done with parents almost two decades ago was limited to the accomplishments of the children, such as whether they could crawl, walk or speak a few words.

Barbara was recently involved in developing and conducting a study of 372 parents who were asked much different questions. Is your child happy? Is your life enriched? What is the effect on your relationship/marriage? On siblings? Describe what your child likes to do. Describe your favourite and most challenging memories. Close to 90 percent of the parents reported a positive, enriching experience with a happy child — a finding Barbara anticipates may cause doctors to pause and to take parents more seriously.

The results of this study were presented at the 2011 meeting of the American Society for Bioethics and Humanities. Barbara explained why she considers this to be the highlight of her advocacy work:

> The room was packed with ethicists and clinicians. I was able to observe the presentations and those watching — something I can't do when I am at the podium. I watched these professionals listening and taking notes as pictures of "our trisomy kids," smiling and laughing, were shown on the screen and quotes by parents were read out loud. After so much work for so many years, it happened.
>
> I am also grateful to the parents who responded to our survey, who either took time out from a busy schedule of caring for a disabled child or who revisited painful but happy memories of their child who had passed away.
>
> With the help of special doctors, I had brought the parents' voice about the love and the value of trisomy kids as well as their beauty to the medical community. Dr. Annie Janvier, one of the doctors with whom I did the research, and I looked at each other and smiled, both of us with tears in our eyes.

A neonatologist with a Ph.D. in bioethics, Dr. Janvier is the mother of a micro-preemie child (born before 26 weeks gestation).

She supports parental autonomy within reason and publishes widely on the devaluation of premature babies as well as many other ethical issues.

Barbara is co-author of the paper "The Experience of Families with Children with Trisomy 13 and 18 in Social Networks," which was published in the journal *Pediatrics*.[1] Publication in such a prestigious journal will assist in bringing the results of this milestone study to the attention of the medical community.

In recognition of the collaborative nature of the study, Barbara said: "I'm so grateful to the many friends, advocates, ethicists and health-care providers who have helped along the way. Special recognition goes to Dr. Ben Wilfond and Dr. Annie Janvier, the co-authors of the paper, who spent a great deal of time over the past two years on an unfunded project simply because they care about children and families and believe that everyone has a right to be heard."

In 2012, Barbara played a key role in establishing the Support Organization for Trisomy International (SOFT International). The organization's mission is to serve all of the trisomy 13 and 18 parental support groups in the world by providing them with accurate information. The original SOFT organization began almost three decades ago in the United States and many chapters were subsequently established around the world.

In Barbara's numerous presentations and papers, she never mentions the name of the hospital where Annie died. She wants people to realize that the type of events that occurred could happen anywhere. Barbara's ability to understand and forgive has allowed her to devote herself entirely to constructive advocacy work.

Barbara's consistent, high-quality work has been recognized in numerous ways, including her appointment as an advisor to the deVeber Institute of Bioethics and Social Research, Toronto, and to the Canadian Patient Safety Institute. She has also been appointed a member of the World Alliance for Patient Safety, Imperial College, London, and the Safe Childbirth Checklist Project, World Health Organization, Geneva.

Barbara has been encouraged by the positive feedback she has received to her insightful, informative and balanced presentations over the years. James B. McCormick, RPT, president of the National Association of Respiratory Therapy Regulators, wrote:

> Her poise, factual, orderly and measured presentation of her family's ordeal, combined with her palpable passion and yet balanced sense of "telling it as it occurred" from her family's perspective left me feeling grateful. Grateful that her audience was not so much reduced to tears, but coaxed to contemplation, reflection and asking both why and how a different process might have enabled a different outcome.
>
> I applaud her ability to lead us through that sad tale whilst challenging our assumptions and prompting us to revisit our corporate platitudes around client-centred care. Having policies on ethics is often quite different than creating a systemic corporate culture that respects the patient/family wishes as central to the delivery of health care.

Barbara's work is having an impact on the next generation of physicians. Below are excerpts from comments made by a student of medicine at McGill University. "Making promises and definitive statements is tantamount to unprofessionalism given our reliance on p-values and error bars and our glorified vagueness of suggestion. Today, I put all that aside. Today, I promise Annie's mom and her husband, and her daughters and her son . . . I shall never treat any patient in any manner that does less than preserve their dignity, pride, honour and humanity. I promise to never stand by and watch colleagues, regardless of their seniority, violate patients or their families and especially those who are most defenceless. I promise to do what I can and, to the best of my ability, to advocate for the humanity in situations where it seems too often lost."

In August 2011, Barbara sent an email to friends and supporters informing them that she and Tim had signed the settlement release for a lawsuit against the hospital. The main reason for their decision was the hospital's revision of a glossary definition of trisomy 13 and 18. Barbara felt that the existing definition led the reader to believe that all children like Annie die soon after birth. The revised definition is consistent with the literature and the definition posted by other leading children's hospitals. The wide spectrum of genetic conditions and the fact that 5 percent to 10 percent of trisomy 13 and 18 babies survive, sometimes into their teens, is now explicitly stated in the glossary definition.

In conclusion, Barbara wrote: "My family loved Annie to the moon and back, without conditions. As long as she could be happy and comfortable, we wanted her to live. To all the very special people on our journey who listened and or who encouraged, supported and advised us, we sincerely thank you. You have given our baby a voice. Annie's message is that love, especially unconditional love, is the greatest quality there is."

Broken

On the night of September 12, 1997, more than 100 teenagers gathered at Stokes Pit, a favourite bush party spot near Surrey, BC. Most were just starting grade 12. As they were saying their goodbyes and getting into their cars to go home, an intoxicated 16-year-old youth driving too fast and passing in and out of consciousness plowed into them. At least 25 students were taken to hospital with serious injuries. Ashley Reber, 17, died instantly. Heidi Klompas, 17, died three and a half weeks later, not from her injuries, but from complications arising from the treatment she received in two hospitals.

This is the story of the events that led to Heidi's death, subsequent investigations and denials of wrongdoing. It tells of the shock Heidi's family suffered when they discovered that in the eyes of the law her life had little value. This is also the story of what Heidi's mother, Catherine Adamson, has done to prevent similar tragedies, with an emphasis on medical care and wrongful death compensation law in British Columbia.

Hospital: September 13 to October 8, 1997

Heidi arrived at Peace Arch District Hospital in White Rock, BC, at 1:29 a.m., approximately 20 minutes after the ambulance left the accident scene. In the emergency room, she was conscious and her vital signs were found to be within the normal range. X-rays revealed multiple severe fractures to both legs below the knee. Both tibia and fibula were jaggedly broken, twisted and overlapping. No other significant injuries were found. Heidi was placed on an intravenous morphine drip for pain. The ER physician called the orthopedic surgeon at 2:30 a.m.

Catherine arrived at the hospital just after 2 a.m. to find Heidi talkative, aware of what happened at the accident scene and in pain. Approximately an hour later, Catherine asked the ER physician when surgery could be done on Heidi's legs. The physician said she had already contacted the orthopedic surgeon half an hour before and that he had said he would be in shortly. The ER physician called the surgeon three more times. After the last call at 7 a.m., when the ER physician was going off shift, she told Catherine the orthopedic surgeon said he would be at the hospital by 9 a.m. to do Heidi's surgery. Catherine asked the nurses if Heidi could be transferred to another hospital where she could have surgery done immediately. The nurses told her the surgery wouldn't be performed any earlier at another hospital.

During the almost seven hours from the time of the first call to the orthopedic surgeon until his arrival at 9:15 a.m., Heidi's legs became increasingly swollen and extremely sensitive to touch. She became groggy and confused, presumably because of the large amount of morphine required to ease her pain.

The surgeon examined Heidi, ordered lateral x-rays of her legs and told Catherine he was going to another hospital to perform a hip operation and would operate on Heidi's legs in the afternoon. The surgeon was concerned about compartment syndrome and told the nurse to check the pulses in Heidi's feet. Acute compartment syndrome is typically associated with some form of trauma, such as fractures, and often occurs in the front compartment of the lower leg. The syndrome develops as a result of swelling or bleeding within a compartment. Because fascia, the layer of fibrous tissue surrounding muscles, does not stretch, pressure is put on the capillaries, nerves and muscles in the compartment, which in turn disrupts blood flow. A characteristic symptom is extreme pain, especially in response to touch. Acute compartment syndrome is a surgical emergency that requires cutting open the skin and fascia covering the affected compartment. This operation is called a fasciotomy.

  The surgeon did not appear to be concerned about the five- to seven-hour delay in surgery. He ordered more morphine for pain control.

Catherine accompanied Heidi when she was taken to the radiology department for the additional x-rays ordered by the surgeon. In Catherine's words: "This new jostling (from being transported on a gurney) caused more pain. Heidi whispered to me, "Mom, it really hurts." I told her to be strong, to just endure the pain for a little while longer until her operation. Heidi promised to be brave for me and tried not to cry. When she said, "I love you, Mom," it sent a shiver up my spine. It sounded too much like a farewell."

Concerned that Heidi's legs had not been properly supported with splints, the x-ray technician did not proceed with taking the lateral x-rays. In particular, the technician was worried that the bones might puncture the taut skin. At 9:40 a.m., while still in the radiology department, Heidi started to have seizures. Medical personnel rushed to her side. Heidi was then taken to the emergency room where there were conflicting reports given about whether or not she had vomited while in the x-ray room.

A neurosurgeon at the Royal Columbian Hospital (RCH) in New Westminster was contacted at 10 a.m. Heidi was placed in a chemically induced coma and transferred by ambulance to the larger hospital, arriving at 11:55 a.m. Catherine stood by her daughter's side in the ER of the Royal Columbian. She recalled:

> I watched as the assisting orthopedic surgeon removed the blanket to expose Heidi's legs. He shouted, "Oh my God, look what they've done to her legs!" Alarmed, I asked him what he meant. He pointed to the tensor bandages that were tightly wound around each ankle, and as he quickly tried to remove them he told me they were cutting off circulation. Heidi could lose the use of both of her feet. I did not fully absorb

this information until the attending orthopedic surgeon agreed with the assisting surgeon and spoke angrily about the Peace Arch doctors who had done this. I was becoming increasingly frightened. These doctors at RCH appeared alarmed. Heidi was still in a coma and her brain was not responding well. Her blood oxygen level was continuing to drop, because her lungs were not functioning properly. Suddenly, her legs were the least of my worries. I was really scared.

Heidi was attended by an emergency room physician, a neurosurgeon and two orthopedic surgeons who conducted examinations and ordered a myriad of tests. A chest x-ray showed congestion and some patchy air spaces in her lungs. A physician suggested that Heidi may have aspirated stomach contents into her lungs. There was no indication of this having occurred on the paperwork from Peace Arch Hospital.

Starting at 3:55 p.m., Heidi underwent surgery (fasciotomy) on her right leg to relieve the compartment syndrome and on both legs to repair the fractures. She was out of surgery at 8:30 p.m. and taken to the post-anaesthetic care unit, where she was monitored carefully, including for the possibility of compartment syndrome developing in the left leg. Shortly afterward, the nurses notified the orthopedic surgeon that they were unable to find a pulse in Heidi's left foot, which was now mottled and discoloured. A few minutes past midnight, early on September 14, the surgeon performed a fasciotomy on Heidi's left leg. She took longer than anticipated to recovery from the anesthetic.

At 7:30 a.m., Heidi was transferred to the intensive care unit (ICU). At the time, she had an elevated temperature, abnormally rapid heartbeat and a lung infection. Physicians began to suspect that Heidi's lung problems were caused by aspiration and fat embolism syndrome. This syndrome is caused by fat globules (emboli) entering the blood stream where they can plug key blood vessels. These emboli can arise from the marrow of fractured bones. The risk of developing this syndrome increases with the number of long bone fractures.

Between the numerous tests conducted on Heidi, Catherine was allowed to see her daughter. She recalled: "I was told I could only spend about five minutes with her. I whispered to her to hang in there, that she'd be okay soon. She didn't respond in any way to my voice. She appeared to be in a deep sleep. I believed it was the drugs that were keeping her under, when in fact it was her brain that was not responding. Later, the neurosurgeon explained that fat from the marrow of Heidi's broken bones had entered her bloodstream and was making contact with her brain and causing a series of mini-strokes that caused her brain to swell."

Five days later, on September 19, Catherine and Heidi's father were awakened by the phone ringing at 3:25 a.m. A physician told them that Heidi was "crashing fast" and they should get to the hospital as soon as possible. In the middle of the conversation, the physician said Heidi had taken a sudden turn for the better. Her intracranial pressure was dropping and she was, according to the physician, "coming back."

As Catherine recalled, "Heidi's father's hand was frozen to the telephone receiver. He was trying to catch his breath as he told me they got her back and that she wasn't going to die right this minute. We were both upright, kneeling on our bed, hyperventilating; both of us were absolutely white in the face and our hearts were hammering in our chests. This was the most frightening phone call of our lives."

The following days and weeks were an emotional roller-coaster ride for Heidi's parents. The high point came on September 26, when a CT scan revealed Heidi's brain to be stable and no additional damage was observed. Catherine said about that day:

> The physician explained the plans for the next day. Heidi would go into surgery and have a tracheostomy to aid in her recovery and to save her vocal cords from damage as she recovered consciousness. The OETT [oral endotracheal tube] had been in her trachea for two weeks now. It passed through her vocal cords and when she woke up she would try to make sounds, and this could cause permanent damage to the cords, hence the need for the tracheostomy. The physician informed me that he would perform the tracheostomy himself, instead of the usual team of specialists who do this type of surgery. He wanted to position the hole lower down on her neck to reduce the visibility of what would surely be

an unsightly scar. He told me he preferred to do most of the tracheostomies on his own patients. I trusted in his judgment as he had saved Heidi's brain, and her life, so far. He and this wonderful team of doctors and nurses had wrestled the seemingly relentless fat embolism beast to the ground and we were getting close to a victory. In addition to the tracheostomy, Heidi was to have her intracranial pressure and external ventricular drains removed.

I couldn't believe this wonderful news! Heidi was definitely improving and the doctors were more optimistic now for a full recovery than they had ever been before. I was so happy.

The next day, September 27, the tracheostomy was performed without incident, but Heidi's intracranial pressure increased during surgery so the drains were left in place. By noon on September 28, Heidi's temperature had increased and her blood pressure decreased. Chest x-rays revealed the tracheostomy tube was in a satisfactory position. However, the x-rays also showed extensive clouding in the left lower lobe of Heidi's lung. At 3 p.m., the tracheostomy site was cleaned again, because it continued to ooze the foul-smelling greyish brown discharge observed earlier in the day. The nurses' notes show that the physician had been made aware of this situation. In the evening, the oxygen level in Heidi's blood dropped.

Although Heidi continued to show worrisome signs for the next week, Catherine had renewed hope for her daughter. Heidi was breathing without assistance and was starting to regain consciousness. She was moved out of the intensive care unit to a maxi ward. Catherine and her husband decided to stay with Heidi in shifts, so the other could attend to neglected duties at home.

Heidi's father visited her for an hour at noon on October 4. Just before leaving at 1 p.m., he noticed the T-piece in her neck was askew. In fact, it was quite crooked and he told the nurse. He watched in surprise as the nurse jerked the T-piece back into position. This rough treatment bothered him. He told Catherine about it later.

After her father left, the nurse heard coarse crackles in Heidi's lungs, so suctioned them, obtaining a moderate amount of yellow secretion. Heidi coughed a little. At 1:50 p.m., the nurse heard Heidi cough again. She immediately checked Heidi and was stunned to see bright red blood spurting out of Heidi's trachea with each cough. The blood was filling the oxygen tubing and blocking the airway. The nurse instantly called for help.

Heidi's parents, who were in separate locations away from the hospital, were notified. Her father arrived first. Catherine's account is this:

> I was met by a doctor in the hallway and he prevented me from entering Heidi's room, which had its doors closed. This doctor ushered me into a small office and, as I was about to enter, I was shocked when I saw a nurse coming out of Heidi's room. Walking with assistance, the nurse was shaking and unsteady on her feet. She was covered in blood. Inside the office, I saw Heidi's father and brother and their faces were ashen. I knew this was going to be bad. The doctor explained what had happened to Heidi, how an artery had burst open and caused a big bleed. He told me her heart had stopped for 20 minutes, and even though they tried to do CPR, he expected that her brain had been irretrievably damaged by this lack of oxygen for a sustained period. He told me she most likely would be brain-dead within a few days. He also said, "We don't keep vegetables alive in our hospital." He told us we should be thinking of organ donation. They would, however, take Heidi into surgery to fix the source of the bleed as soon as it could be arranged. At this point, he said he didn't know exactly what happened, but surgery would give more details.

Two days later, October 6, the neurosurgeon spoke in detail with Catherine. He had examined the CT scan taken after the traumatic bleed. He was visibly shaken. However, he remained hopeful that the CPR that was performed would have supplied the minimum amount of oxygen to save most of Heidi's brain. If she survived, she might be blinded or at least have diminished eyesight. He told Catherine that if blindness was the only damage, the family should feel lucky.

Catherine spent most of the following day with Heidi. She

underwent more tests, including another CT scan. The crackling sound when she breathed continued to be evident.

Close to 3:30 p.m., there occurred what Catherine describes as a brief, soul-altering moment of absoluteness for her: "As I was looking at Heidi, she suddenly opened her eyes wide and stared straight at me and I felt this great rush of foreign energy pass through me like an invisible splash. It is hard to describe. I thought to myself, 'Oh God, no!' It's as if Heidi was telling me goodbye, that she would be going now. I held my breath and thought, 'This is it, I'm really losing her.' I kept talking to her, but she was no longer responding."

After waiting into the evening to see the neurosurgeon, Catherine drove home. Upon arrival, her husband told her that the neurosurgeon had called to say Heidi was brain-dead. Not wanting to believe what she heard, Catherine called the neurosurgeon, who told her the CT scan showed massive brain damage and Heidi was not showing any signs of neurological activity. He said there was absolutely no hope. On October 8, tests confirmed brain-death, and on October 9, Heidi was taken to the operating room for organ retrieval. Her heart, liver and kidneys gave four people renewed hope for life. Her corneas gave two other people the gift of vision.

Investigations, Lawsuit and Altered Lives

An autopsy performed on October 15, 1997, at Royal Columbian Hospital found the immediate cause of death was anoxic (lack of oxygen) brain injury as a result of massive blood loss from erosion of the innominate artery as a result of pressure from a tracheostomy tube. The innominate artery, also known as the brachiocephalic artery, supplies blood to the right arm, head and neck.

A proximal cause of death was complications of treatments as a result of having been struck by a motor vehicle while a pedestrian and included multiple blunt force injuries and long bone fractures resulting in fat emboli syndrome.

In January 1998, the BC Coroners Service began a thorough investigation into Heidi's death. A coroner's investigation presents facts only, does not lay blame and may make non-binding recommendations. The report, which was released in July 1999, was based on examination of medical records, interviews with Catherine and medical personnel and relevant articles in medical books and journals.

The ER physician at Peace Arch Hospital confirmed to the coroner that she notified the on-call orthopedic surgeon several times during the early hours of September 13. In contrast, the surgeon said he was almost 99 percent certain he was not notified more than one time. Although he recognized the early signs of compartment syndrome, the surgeon thought there was no real urgency.

Citing papers in medical journals, the coroner wrote that the best treatment for fat embolism syndrome is prevention, which consists of early fixation of long bone fractures. Also, full attention should be paid to preventive measures, which include minimizing movement of the fractured bones and splinting at the earliest possibility opportunity. Early immobilization is known to have a positive influence on reducing the incidence of the syndrome. Heidi's legs were not properly splinted until she was at the Royal Columbian Hospital, more than 12 hours after they had been broken.

The coroner wrote that although Heidi suffered from significant morbidity as a result of fat embolism syndrome, she was on the path to recovery in that her pneumonia was resolving and her neurological functioning was improving. Heidi's death was caused by anoxic brain injury sustained from a cardiac arrest caused by the rupture of the innominate artery from a fistula. This fistula, or abnormal passage, between the trachea and the innominate artery had not been diagnosed until the hemorrhage and cardiac arrest occurred.

The location of the tracheostomy incision was an important factor. Considering how self-conscious a teenage girl would be about a scar on her neck, the surgeon placed the incision lower than is recommended. This well-intentioned decision had deadly consequences, as the tracheostomy was close enough to the innominate artery to allow for development of a fistula. This perforation of the arterial wall resulted in the large hemorrhage, which in turn led to cerebral anoxia.

The coroner recommended that Peace Arch Hospital conduct

educational rounds on the treatment and risks associated with serious fractures and that the Royal Columbian Hospital do a similar exercise regarding the risks associated with the placement of tracheostomy tubes.

In due course, a physician at the Royal Columbian wrote to the chief coroner: "In summary, therefore, careful review of this unfortunate lady's care at Royal Columbian Hospital does not identify any measures or any modification of medical management which could be reasonably assumed to have changed her clinical course."

Catherine visited the ICU at the Royal Columbian several weeks after Heidi's funeral to thank the nurses for the care they had given her daughter. In conversation with the head nurse of the ICU, Catherine mentioned the fistula and hemorrhage. The nurse said how sorry she was, and that she and other nurses knew about fistulas but hadn't thought to check for one in Heidi's situation.

The Children's Commission Fatality Review report, done independently from the coroner's report, came to similar conclusions. Released in January 2000, the report contained two recommendations directed at the College of Physicians and Surgeons of British Columbia. These were for the College to review the medical care provided to Heidi with reference to the delay in examination by an orthopedic surgeon and to review the procedure followed during surgery for the placement of a tracheostomy tube.

Having seen the evidence of possible medical malpractice in both the coroner's and Fatality Review reports, Catherine wrote to the College herself with specific questions about Heidi's care. She also asked the College to consider the impact on family members of the words of the physician who had told her they don't "keep vegetables alive in their hospital." When questioned by the College, the physician denied using the term "vegetable." Several of Heidi's family members, in addition to Catherine, had heard the doctor say the word.

Nine months later, Catherine received a 10-page letter from the College dated December 15, 2000. The College's summary is as follows: "it was the committee's opinion that Heidi suffered a tragic accident on the highway, and received appropriate emergency care. She then had the misfortune to suffer a significant and severe fat embolism to the brain, which led to significant brain damage. Subsequently she had the further misfortune to suffer an uncommon complication of her tracheostomy which led to a massive bleed from the innominate artery in the neck, which was followed by a prolonged period of cardiac arrest, resulting in further brain damage from which it was impossible to recover." In other words, the College did not find fault with any part of Heidi's care.

An in-depth investigation by Rick Ouston that appeared in the *Vancouver Sun* on November 11, 2000 reported that the orthopedic surgeon in question at Peace Arch Hospital had lost four negligence suits and settled two others out of court. Two other claims of negligence were filed against him in the late 1990s, but neither was pursued. A hospital other than Peace Arch had three times relieved the surgeon of his privileges to practice at the hospital. He went to court and got his privileges restored. In 1993, the College struck the surgeon's name from the permanent register of physicians. He was placed on the temporary register and ordered to receive psychotherapy. Two years later, he was returned to the permanent register.

Catherine retained a lawyer to handle the family's claim with the Insurance Corporation of British Columbia (ICBC). After receiving the two government reports, she considered launching a medical malpractice lawsuit. Her lawyer advised against it for a number of reasons, not the least of which was provincial laws pertaining to the death of a child. In Catherine's words:

> Because Heidi's injuries began with a car crash, ICBC had to be the initial focus of a claim for loss. If we wanted to sue for malpractice, then we would have to include everyone all at once, because BC laws do not permit anyone to sue more than once for the same death. Therefore, we would have to sue the hospital, all the doctors and nurses involved and the ICBC together in one lawsuit. This would have been a huge undertaking and the legal fees could have cost at least $200,000. The expected compensation was less than $50,000, which would mean we might stand to lose a minimum of $150,000.

We were not a wealthy family and could not afford such a staggering financial loss. Nevertheless, I pressured my lawyer to go forward mostly because I wanted the public to know what really happened to Heidi in the hospitals. He directed me to a large firm in Vancouver that dealt with malpractice suits: after discussing Heidi's case with me, their lawyer confirmed what my lawyer had said: a malpractice suit was not feasible unless I would be able to spend hundreds of thousands of dollars and five to 10 years just to make my point. Defeated, I agreed to go ahead with the single lawsuit against ICBC.

In monetary terms, a child's life is virtually worthless in Canada. The BC legal guidelines for death of a child come from the Family Compensation Act, and the amounts recoverable are usually for medical costs, funeral costs and the loss of income we would have expected from our daughter had she gone on to earn a living for the rest of her life while supporting us. Obviously, this is negligible, as we never expected our children to support us. There is no compensation allowable for the pain and suffering of parents when they lose a child. There is no compensation for the marriages that fall apart after the death of a child. I read once that the divorce rate is as high as 75 percent for couples who have lost a child. Our marriage succumbed and joined this sad majority within a year. The loss of half my husband's income (as an airline pilot) was not a consideration for compensation by ICBC's lawyer. In addition to everything else, I was unable to continue to work as a realtor and relinquished my licence during the first year.

Two days before Christmas in 1999, ICBC offered Heidi's family a settlement of $5,000. They refused and over the next 18 months offers and counteroffers were sent between the lawyers. Finally, all parties agreed to go to mediation. Catherine recalled:

I did not see my day in court where I had hoped to tell the world (through the media) all that my daughter endured. In August of 2001, nearly four years after Heidi's death, we settled the claim in mediation. We signed a non-disclosure agreement with ICBC, and therefore I am not permitted to disclose the amount we received. Just let me say that the amount I personally received was far less than $100,000. At that point, I was a single woman going to university. The money allowed me to repay my parents for the down payment on my little house, pay off my car loan and almost pay off the credit card debt. I was penniless, but oh so relieved that the years of bickering with ICBC were over.

Our courts and our lawmakers need to take a broader look at the actual damages a family suffers after the death of a child. In Heidi's case, the two government investigations clearly pointed to medical errors and omissions as the cause of her death. Where was the apology? The emotional toll on us had been huge. Bill and Laura (Heidi's brother and sister) each lost three years of schooling. I lost my marriage, my security, my spark. I am forever a changed woman. Some viable financial security at this time in my life would have been most welcome.

I feel there should be two ways of calculating compensation to victims. Certainly people should be reimbursed for costs incurred, but I feel there should also be larger awards given as deterrents for those who harm. The courts should charge the doctors and hospitals amounts that exceed their comfort zones. Currently, doctors in BC are virtually untouchable. Our legal system is set up to allow them to harm, even to the point of causing death, with impunity. This is wrong and this system must be changed to better protect patients and their families.

In 1999, Catherine returned to university. Over the next four years she earned a Bachelor of Arts degree in English and Visual Arts from the University College of the Fraser Valley. In 2005, she returned to Vancouver, her birthplace, where she continues to write and paint. While at university, Catherine accumulated the documentation required to tell Heidi's story.

The Book: *Heidi Dawn Klompas: Missed Opportunities*

In 2005, Catherine published *Heidi Dawn Klompas: Missed Opportunities* based on over 800 pages of hospital records, research papers and reports, and her own memories. She wrote the book for a number of reasons, including that nurses and doctors might better understand why they should pay closer attention to the concerns of the parents of their patients. In addition, she wanted the College of Physicians and Surgeons of British Columbia to review their mandate to protect the public. Catherine also hoped that Canadians might see themselves in the ordinary people in her book and realize "this too could happen to their families."

Writing a book is akin to skipping stones on water. You know you will create waves, but you don't know their number, their size or what their impact will be. In an email dated November 28, 2011, Catherine told of two particular gratifying impacts of her book.

When I completed my book, I went to all the Vancouver-area hospitals and left a few copies in doctors' and nurses' lounges. I also handed the book to anyone I saw in scrubs, hoping to reach as many surgeons as possible. That was in 2006.

Years later, a friend, Robert, told me a wonderful story. He had been in a car accident two years before our conversation and had broken many bones, both large and small. He was taken to Vancouver General Hospital's emergency room where a doctor hooked him up to an IV and then gave him an injection of an anti-clotting drug. Robert asked him what the drug was for and the surgeon said it was to reduce the chance of clots hitting his brain, because they didn't want another Klompas on their hands. Robert asked him if he meant Heidi Klompas. Surprised the surgeon said, "Yes. How do you know about her?" Robert told him he knew Heidi's mother and that she had written a book about what happened to Heidi. The surgeon said that he and his colleagues had all read the book and that was why Robert was getting the drug — to prevent the same thing from happening again. When Robert told me this, I was astounded. I am so pleased that my book is helping to save lives, as that was the original purpose of writing it.

The head of curriculum for the University of British Columbia's Medical School read my book. She is now incorporating parts of it into the current curriculum and hopes to use the entire book within the next few years. Right now, it's in the five libraries UBC has for medical students across the province. I find this encouraging.

Wrongful Death Law Reform Group

In 2006, Catherine joined the Wrongful Death Law Reform Group (WDLRG). The group consists of more than 50 families who work with other organizations (BC Coalition of People with Disabilities, Trial Lawyers Association of BC and the Coalition Against No-Fault) to bring about a Wrongful Death Accountability Act. This act contains an integrated series of statutory reforms designed to ensure that the two goals of fair compensation and meaningful deterrence are satisfied in every situation where a person is killed by the negligent conduct of another. In the view of the WDLRG, this act provides solutions to the weak and unfair law currently in place, the Family Compensation Act, which is based on legislation originating in the United Kingdom in 1846. The British law disallows damages for lost love, guidance, care, companionship and affection.

In conjunction with the group, Catherine has written letters to politicians and attended meetings. She also included Heidi's story in the WDLRG's anthology of real-life stories of wrongful deaths. This anthology, *In Their Name*, was submitted to the Ministry of the Attorney General of British Columbia in 2008. A year later, Heidi's story formed part of a related video, *Wrongful Death Reform*. In September 2011, Catherine joined with approximately 60 other people who gathered on the steps of the Vancouver Art Gallery to rally for change to the Family Compensation Act.

The Media

Heidi's story attracted considerable media attention at the time of her death, later with the release of the coroner's report and again when Catherine discovered she would not receive compensation for her daughter's death. Catherine made herself available to reporters whenever possible. She wrote two particularly poignant letters to the editor of the *Vancouver Sun*. In a letter dated October 10, 1997, she expressed sympathy for the intoxicated youth who had struck the students. "We have no anger. No hard feelings toward this family. It's just a tragedy all the way around," she wrote. On May 5, 1999, what would have been Heidi's 19th birthday, Catherine wrote a letter shaming the unknown man who had purchased beer for the later-to-be-intoxicated youth.

Catherine was instrumental in ensuring that local police check the alcohol level of all drivers when breaking up large parties of young people. She was also a member of Mothers Against Drunk Drivers for several years.

A Doctor's Ordeal

When Jacques Besson, a retired French physician, checked into a Montreal hospital in August 2003 for surgery on a herniated disc, he anticipated a rapid recovery free of complications. That had been his experience when he had undergone the same surgery 15 years before in France. Instead, Besson, at age 83, spent almost a year fighting for his life in a battle against multiple hospital-acquired infections. The experience turned Besson into a leading advocate for safer, cleaner hospitals. In 2004, Besson, his daughter, Christine Besson, and friends founded the Association for the Defense of Victims of Nosocomial Infections (ADVIN), which was later renamed Association for Victims of Nosocomial Infection. Advocacy work was a new venture for the retired doctor. In his 45-year medical career in France, he had dedicated himself to his patients, teaching courses in a faculty of medicine and helping to found the French Association of Allergists. Besson and his wife, Eglantine Porte, moved to Montreal in 1995 to spend their later years with their children and grandchildren. Christine, now a retired high school principal, was at her father's side throughout his illness. She continues to play a key role in raising public and professional awareness of the impact of nosocomial infections and what can be done to reduce their staggering impact in suffering, loss of life and financial cost. Each year, 220,000 to 250,000 hospital-acquired infections result in 8,000 to 12,000 deaths in Canada. Most of these infections are preventable.

In addition to causing immense human suffering and loss of life, hospital-acquired infections take an enormous financial toll. It's estimated that their annual cost in the United States is US$30 billion; in France, US$8 billion; and in Quebec, more than US$180 million. Canadian researchers estimate that the total attributable cost to treat MRSA infections is $14,360 per patient. The total cost of HAIs in Canada easily approaches $3 billion, and there are many thousands of such patients each year. These infections also worsen waiting lists by extending the duration of hospitalization. Simple, inexpensive measures to combat these infections have repeatedly been shown to be effective in Europe, the United States and Canada. With an investment of only $200,000 in a hand hygiene campaign, the LeGardeur Hospital in Lanaudière, near Montreal, reduced the number of MRSA infections by 500 cases over a five-year period with a savings of $1.5 million.

Infection

At home three days after surgery, Jacques Besson developed excruciating pain, sweating and chills. Six days later, after being seen at the emergency room of another hospital and with considerable pressure from his daughter, he was readmitted to the hospital where surgery had been performed. Staff determined Besson's increasingly severe symptoms were a result of infection of the surgical site.

Two weeks later, Besson underwent a second surgery to clean the wound. Laboratory tests showed he had multiple bacterial infections, including methicillin-resistant *Staphylococcus aureus* (MRSA), a "superbug" that kills thousands of patients annually. By this time, Besson was suffering intense pain from the infections, which had spread to his abdomen and thigh. He repeatedly told his family that he wanted to die.

In mid-November, Besson's infection was considered to be under control and he was sent home even though he was continuing to experience intense pain. The following day, his fever spiked and Christine was forced to resort to threatening the surgeon in order to have her father admitted to hospital the same day. Besson continued to endure significant pain and underwent intensive antibiotic treatment.

To compound his misery, Besson acquired *Clostridium difficile*, a bacterium that causes severe diarrhea. This scourge was responsible for the deaths of nearly 2,000 patients in 2003 and 2004 in Quebec alone.

At the beginning of December, following extensive treatment for pain, Besson went into such a deep narcoleptic sleep for 36 hours that the doctors thought he was dying.

Within a few weeks, Besson had recovered from the C. *difficile* infection. The surgeon's assistant told him that the MRSA infection was under control and that, consequently, he was being released from hospital. Christine described the situation and subsequent events.

> My father and I were very skeptical of the "under control" diagnosis, considering his pain level and general state. But I could not get anything else from the surgeon's assistant. Since my father's third readmission to hospital in November, I had constantly questioned the surgeon's decisions. Since then, she never visited my father, always sending an assistant.
>
> Ready to leave the hospital, my father was visited by the microbiology resident who was responsible for prescribing the medications for him to take home. This young man declared that my father could not leave and the infection was far from being under control. He had reached this conclusion after taking the time — two hours — to read my father's file.
>
> We were desperate, but at the same time, the resident's diagnosis confirmed our own impression. All through his hospitalization, my father was able to follow the diagnosis and treatments. He was often flabbergasted by the conclusions reached and explanations given by some of the doctors.

Finally, just before Christmas, the resident sent Besson home with a prescription for Vancomycin to be injected daily for 10 weeks. In hospital, the infected surgical site had been placed under a negative pressure machine to accelerate healing. Treatment with this machine was to be continued for two months at home.

A nurse came every day for those two months to inject the Vancomycin and change the special dressing. For the following three months, she came every two to three days. Besson returned to the hospital for checkups and scans every four weeks.

At the end of June, 10 months after surgery, he was finally free of infection. Christine and Besson estimate that during this time he had at least 19 CT scans plus x-rays and innumerable other tests. Reflecting on that difficult time, Christine said: "We were very disappointed by the surgeon's attitude and response to the infection, although the surgery had been a success. In stark contrast, we consider the chief nurse and his main assistant to have saved my father's life. They constantly fought for better painkillers, faster access to scans and other tests, and access to the doctors in person. Often new treatments were given to my father without any explanation or even a visit from the doctor; they just consulted the latest results and prescribed. The importance of the high quality of listening and caring by the nursing staff cannot be overstated. Many times, these people called me at home to inform me that I should come to the hospital to check what was going on."

Before leaving the hospital in December 2003, Besson met with the complaints and quality care commissioner of the hospital. Subsequently, he and Christine sent a letter to the hospital board in charge of medical care. The letter outlined their concerns about his care and requested clarification. Almost a year later, they received a letter which essentially said that all treatments were appropriate and there was no evidence of error.

The suffering of the Besson family was compounded by the death of Eglantine in late July. While her husband was struggling with multiple infections, Eglantine gradually succumbed to complications following a severe bout of pneumonia two years previous.

Public and Professional Education, ADVIN and Wash Your Hands

At the end of August 2004, Besson and Christine consulted with lawyer Jean-Pierre Ménard, whose Montreal office specializes in medical error cases. They were seeking information on the possibility of bringing legal action against the hospital, not with the intent of obtaining money, but to clarify what happened to Besson. In his opinion, the hospital had been negligent in various ways, including in its communication with him. After carefully reviewing Besson's file, Ménard said it would be impossible to sue the hospital, because lines of responsibility could not be clearly established.

Besson, Christine and friends subsequently began exploring the possibility of funding an association to advocate for hospital-acquired infection (HAI) victims. Ménard gave the group his support, including the suggestion that some C. *difficile* victims who were part of a potential class-action suit might be interested in joining the association. A press conference was held at Ménard's office to announce the launch of the class-action suit and the creation of the Association for the Defense of Victims of Nosocomial Infection (ADVIN).

A non-profit organization, ADVIN is run by volunteers and financed by members' fees, donations and public funding from the Ministry of Health Programs for Community Associations. ADVIN's mission is to raise awareness and inform the public about the dangers of HAIs. The association welcomes collaboration with all health, political and professional authorities in order to develop programs of prevention and control of HAIs in accordance with international standards. ADVIN supports victims of these infections and all other patients by informing them of their rights, and it is working toward a compensation plan for victims.

ADVIN is governed by dedicated board members, most of whom have had experience with HAIs. Besson serves as president of the association and Christine as secretary to the board. Christine is also responsible for most of the association's communication, keeping the websites up to date and assisting her father in a variety of ways.

Claude Dumaine, vice-president, was the owner of a garage in Montreal until he broke his leg in 2001. During surgery to repair the fracture, he was infected with MRSA. Dumaine's nightmare is ongoing. The infection in his leg is still not cured and he continues to experience significant pain. He must return almost weekly to hospital for various treatments. Being a member of ADVIN is for Dumaine an opportunity to fight not only for the cause, but for his very life.

A drama coordinator at a Montreal high school, Christian Sénéchal joined ADVIN because committing himself to social causes is part of his personal value system. He has served as treasurer of the board and is now a part-time general manager.

Other board members include Sophie Mongeon, a young lawyer whose father died at 56 as a result of an infection with C. *difficile*, and Ronald Devito, who survived a bout with C. *difficile* after being in a coma for two weeks. Devito's family was told he would die. He is president of a medical insurance company he founded in 1992 that specializes in collective medical insurance.

Board member Jean Thouin founded an association more than 20 years ago aimed at helping patients in their relationship with health and social systems at all levels. Thouin explained why he works with ADVIN: "I joined ADVIN because I firmly believe that citizens become empowered when they associate with each other and that their involvement is the best way to improve our society. Health care centres must take into account their clientele, the patients, if they really want to improve the quality of their services and make them more human."

The board is assisted by two expert committees. The scientific committee is composed of professionals with expertise in microbiology, public health and epidemiology. The communications committee includes experts in web design and other types of communication.

ADVIN's informative websites in both French and English are major contributors to informing the public about HAIs. At the top of each page is a quote from Florence Nightingale that is as applicable today was it was more than 160 years ago: "It may seem a strange principle to enunciate as the very first requirement in a hospital that it should do the sick no harm."

In the first few years of its existence, the association's website received 4,000 visits a month. After a few years, that number levelled off to several hundred visits each month. This decrease is likely a result of a combination of the lessening of the C. *difficile* epidemic in Quebec hospitals and the increase in number of websites providing similar information because of the overall increase in HAIs in Western countries.

The extensive website includes international news articles and global alerts on nosocomial infections and links to relevant worldwide organizations and networks such as the MRSA survivors' network. A particular strength of the website is its up-to-date information. Articles are usually posted within days of appearing in popular or specialized publications.

Vistors to the website learn that every year in Quebec 90,000 people are afflicted by HAIs. More Quebeckers die every year from HAIs than from car accidents and breast cancer combined. An eight-minute video shows how easily C. difficile could be controlled if only there was the will to do so. Website visitors can also learn how to protect themselves during a stay in a hospital. It's particularly important that patients and their families ask staff and visitors to wash their hands, insist that rooms be properly cleaned and request an immediate transfer if sharing a room with an infected person. The website also has personal testimonies and specialized documentation on risk management and the costs and benefits of preventative measures.

Christine reads all the literature on HAIs in French and English and posts information on the websites. Much of Besson's time is spent writing articles and preparing presentations he makes at conferences to give the patient's perspective. He consistently emphasizes the prevention of and socio-economic costs of HAIs. In spite of age and lingering pain, Besson continues to be an active participant in conferences, seminars and courses. A few days shy of his 90th birthday in February 2011, Besson spoke at the introduction of a new master's degree program (QUEOPS) combining health administration and public health at the University of Montreal, in partnership with the French National Public Health School.

In fall 2010, ADVIN launched a Wash Your Hands campaign, which includes a French-only website, lavetesmains.net. The purposes of the campaign are twofold: to inform the public about the critical importance of hand washing in the prevention of infections and to create a network of all the positive initiatives for the prevention and control of HAIs.

The role of physicians' dirty hands in the spread of disease within hospitals was first recognized in 1845 by a Viennese physician, Dr. Ignaz Semmelweiss. It is almost inconceivable that today, more than 165 years later, there is still a need to convince health-care workers to wash their hands. However, such is sadly the case. It has been estimated that 80 percent of nosocomial infections are transmitted by the hands of caregivers. Simple hand washing alone can decrease this by 50 percent.

The Wash Your Hands campaign was successful in attracting the interest of hospitals and health-care centres. During Patient Safety Week in November 2010, ADVIN worked with staff and patients at the hospital in Argenteuil, Quebec, to educate them about the risks of nosocomial infections and how to prevent them. Considerable emphasis was placed on hand hygiene. Patient Safety Week is organized by the Canadian Patient Safety Institute in conjunction with health-care facilities and organizations. In European, American and Canadian hospitals in which hand hygiene campaigns have been undertaken, there has been a consistent and significant reduction in the rate of HAIs.

ADVIN currently is working with another association, le Conseil pour la Protection des Patients, to pursue their common goal of pressuring health authorities to adopt a policy of making public the HAI rates in hospitals and health centres. In addition, ADVIN is working to have other associations, such as the Coalition Priorité Cancer du Québec, join in this work. As ADVIN board member Jean Thouin said, the association of empowered citizens is the best way to improve society, including health care.

Christine explained that this is a complex goal: "Ideally we'd like to see the obligatory declaration of all HAI infections in a no-fault system with financial compensation for victims. It is a complex matter involving legal aspects such as the definition of an HAI and hospital responsibility and liability. We're emphasizing that the solution to the HAI problem is better management, not finding culprits. As for patients, they are now left alone when they find themselves crippled or sick for months without any resource or support from the hospital where infection occurred."

Other countries have obligatory reporting systems for hospitals. In France, members of the public can find the rate of infectious diseases in their local hospital on the web. To promote transparency, many American states require hospitals to publicly report their infection rates. These and other proposed initiatives by professional and government bodies give ADVIN hope for change in Quebec.

Besson, Christine and other members of ADVIN are exploring the possibility of holding a conference focused on promising new approaches to combat HAIs. The proposed conference would facilitate an integrated approach to this complex problem by bringing together health professionals, caregivers, health managers, hospital administrators, patient associations and partners from the health industry. To bring this project to fruition requires the dedication of a small number of professionals and financial support.

The Canada Revenue Agency does not consider ADVIN a charitable organization because it advocates for change, which is considered a political action. Funding for all of its activities is a continuing challenge for the association. Much of the routine work is done on a volunteer basis. In general, ADVIN has been well received by government and professional groups. Several provided letters of support for the Wash Your Hands campaign. The Quebec Ministry of Health through the public health department provided most of the funds for the campaign. Recently, ADVIN received a letter from the Quebec Committee on Nosocomial Infections offering support for the proposed conference on integrated management. The reluctance of some scientific and medical specialists to support the campaign, apparently out of fear of potential legal action, is changing.

Reflecting on her father's long career and changes in medicine, Christine said:

> The association [ADVIN] is a perfect continuation of my father's interest
> in medicine. When he started practicing, antibiotics had just come into

widespread use[1] and infectious diseases were the main killers in hospitals. Hygiene was strict and diagnosis was based on clinical symptoms and questions. The relationship between the physician and his patient was very important and based on human aspects as well as scientific considerations. There were very few diagnostic tests at the time. In his lifetime, my father has witnessed tremendous scientific discoveries and improvements in medical techniques and treatments. Scientific medicine triumphed and doctors basked in the glory.

My father's confrontation with a tough infection also confronted him with the consequences or collateral aspects of this modern, extremely scientific and technical medicine: patients considered as a collection of different parts and not as a whole person, doctors taking care of the disease but not of the patient, and lack of communication with patients and between specialists . . . and at the far end the patient lost in his bed. Risk of bacterial infection brings us back to basics. Do no harm. The patient must be the centre of care.

Special Recognition

The day after Terence Young's 15-year-old daughter, Vanessa, suddenly died, March 19, 2000, he began his journey to find out why. Questions and comments by attending medical professionals led him to suspect that Prepulsid, which Vanessa had been prescribed for mild bulimia and bloating, had played a role, and that he and Vanessa's mother had not been told the whole story about the drug's known dangerous, even lethal, side effects. Terence spent long hours in his study. He searched the internet for everything he could find about Prepulsid, prescription drugs and the companies that make them. He researched company and government policies regarding testing, warnings and monitoring once the drugs were on the market. He spoke with hundreds of medical and scientific experts. He filled stacks of binders with notes and research papers. On occasion, he left his study to spend time in libraries and also to meet face to face with people who could shed light on why Vanessa died.

Strengthened with a formidable amount of disturbing knowledge, Terence successfully argued for an inquest into the circumstances associated with Vanessa's death. He established the research and advocacy organization Drug Safety Canada (drugsafetycanada.com), launched lawsuits and wrote the book Death by Prescription *(2005), an investigative journey into the world of "Big Pharma."*

"Throughout this book, and through the inspiring work of his

organization, Drug Safety Canada, Terence Young honours his daughter but he also offers hope to the other Canadians harmed by the secrecy and profit mongering that surrounds drug development today," wrote Dr. Nancy Olivieri, Professor, Pediatrics and Medicine, University of Toronto.

To help raise awareness of the dangers associated with prescription drugs, Terence has spoken at conferences and universities and to community groups and the media across the country. He stood by other families who lost children as a result of prescription medications. In 2008, he ran successfully for Member of Provincial Parliament (MPP) for Oakville, Ontario, in order to influence federal regulation of prescription drugs. Respected for his integrity and courage, he was re-elected in May 2011.

Tragedy, Questions and Realization

As Terence Young said, there wasn't much that made his family different from any other, except for their many blessings. Terence and his wife, Gloria, and their three children, Madeline, Vanessa and Hart, lived in Oakville, Ontario, an attractive community with good schools and a low crime rate. A manager with Bell Canada from 1981 to 1994, Terence was elected to the Parliament of Ontario in 1995. He made the news for his private member's bill titled "An Act to Promote Zero Tolerance for Substance Abuse by Children." Four years later, his riding of Halton Centre was eliminated when the number of provincial ridings was reduced. The next year, when the Young family's life changed forever, Terence was building a consultancy business and Gloria was working in public affairs for a hospital.

On a Saturday evening in mid-March 2000, Vanessa, 15, went downstairs to greet her father, who was reading the newspaper in his study. He and Gloria had been out shopping and returned home around 6 p.m., tired and hungry. Terence remembers that Vanessa wanted to ask him something. Suspecting her request had to do with her curfew, he said, "Not now, Vanessa," preferring to delay the discussion until he'd had dinner and was in a better frame of mind.

As Vanessa started to go upstairs, she fell backward, striking the back of her head on the carpet. Terence rushed to his daughter and found her limp, motionless and pale. The possibility that Vanessa had suffered a fainting spell flashed through his mind, but she had never fainted before. In the following few minutes, an ambulance was called, Terence's brother Ted, a surgeon, was contacted and a neighbour, Anna, a registered nurse, came to help Terence with CPR and mouth-to-mouth resuscitation.

Soon Terence was telling the paramedics and an attending police officer that Vanessa's only medication was Prepulsid, which had been prescribed for bloating. She wouldn't have taken any other medication and never used recreational drugs. "She was fine today. She was baking cookies. She probably ate some of them. Nothing like this has ever happened before," Terence told the paramedics. In a search of Vanessa's room and personal items, Gloria and Terence found no drugs other than the prescribed Prepulsid, not even Aspirin or Tylenol.

In hospital, hope flickered briefly when Vanessa's heart began to beat after she had been technically dead for almost half an hour. In the middle of the night, lying exhausted on a couch in the intensive care waiting room, Terence realized there would be no miracle for Vanessa. Too much time had elapsed with her heart being stopped, and then there were the looks on the doctors' faces and their careful choice of words. Vanessa died on Sunday, March 19, 2000, at 1:12 p.m.

In Terence's words: "Why did this happen? I had to find the answer. I began my search the day after Vanessa died."

Questions about Prepulsid (the trade name for the drug cisapride) began in the emergency room. Who had prescribed it? Why did the cardiologist who had revived Vanessa's heart tell Terence, "They dish it [Prepulsid] out like water." Who were "they"? Why were the doctors referring to a large blue book called the *Compendium of Pharmaceuticals and Specialities*? The doctors said that Prepulsid was a dangerous drug for some patients. Something to do with "long QT," which Terence didn't understand. Terence became suspicious that Prepulsid might have played a role in his daughter's death and that he wasn't being told the whole story.

I am not unworldly. I'd been in business for 25 years, and had been a member of the Provincial Parliament for four years. I knew that people make mistakes. I knew they try to cover them up. But this was simply unbelievable.

We were fully aware of Vanessa starting on Prepulsid. No one had cautioned us in any way. If they had, we wouldn't have let her take it. There was simply no reason I could imagine why Vanessa should have fallen down dead. It wasn't just the bleak sadness of Vanessa's death that haunted me. The truth is I had come face to face with a startling truth: even when you try your utmost to protect the ones you love, unseen things can put them in danger. The optimism I had enjoyed for as long as I had known had been supplanted with fear.

That Monday morning I slumped over my desk, head in my hands, playing back the previous two days' events — like rewinding a movie. Tears came without control.

Why Did Vanessa Die?

The first thing Terence wanted to do after Vanessa's death was to warn others about any dangers associated with the use of Prepulsid. Before visiting the funeral home to arrange for Vanessa's funeral, he called Johnson & Johnson's Canadian drug division, Janssen-Ortho in Toronto, which sold Prepulsid in Canada. Terence wanted to tell them what had happened, so they could issue an urgent public warning, and he wanted to ask how on earth this could have happened. What he learned from those phone conversations and the internet was stunning.

Prepulsid was sold worldwide in 119 countries, and U.S. news sources claimed that 341 adverse reactions as well as 80 deaths had been reported from this "heartburn drug." In conversation with a representative of Janssen-Ortho, Terence realized that he wasn't telling the company anything it hadn't known for years. He also came to understand that "the blame game" was on. Janssen had faxed four letters to doctors and there had been two warnings in the *Canadian*

Medical Association Journal concerning risks associated with Prepulsid. It would not be the company's fault that Vanessa died, but rather the fault of her physician, who prescribed Prepulsid and either didn't see or didn't appreciate the significance of the warnings. Terence recalled:

> But Vanessa had seen three other doctors in the previous 14 months. Our gastroenterologist had seen Vanessa in January to test for any blockage in her digestive system that might make her bloated and throw up after meals. A little over a year before, Vanessa had gone to see a psychiatrist for advice on how to deal with her bloated feeling and off-and-on problem of throwing up after meals. And in the previous few weeks, Vanessa had seen a specialist in child psychology twice to talk about it.
>
> Presumably these four doctors had been sent form letters from Prepulsid's manufacturers outlining any dangers.
>
> Neither Gloria nor I had ever been told, however, of any potential risks.

Soon Terence would learn that the dangers associated with Prepulsid had been known for years. A 1992 World Health Organization study raised concerns about the drug. In July 1996, the *Canadian Adverse Drug Reaction Newsletter*[1,2], a quarterly Health Canada publication that appears on the department's website and in the *Canadian Medical Association Journal*,[2] carried a report noting that "serious ventricular arrhythmias" had been observed in some patients taking the drugs who had pre-existing heart problems or risk factors for arrhythmia.

Also in 1996, the Vancouver General Hospital's *Drug and Therapeutics Newsletter*[2] warned doctors to use caution when prescribing Prepulsid to patients with a history of arrhythmia, cardiac disease or electrolyte imbalance.

In late June 1998, the U.S. Food and Drug Administration (FDA) sent a letter to American doctors warning about the danger of an irregular heartbeat associated with Prepulsid.

As of September 16, 1999, Health Canada had received 127 reports of adverse reactions associated with Prepulsid. Seventy of these were of a serious nature, including 35 reports involving heart rate and rhythm disorders. There were 12 reports of fatalities associated with the use of Prepulsid. In the same January 2000 *Adverse Drug Reaction Newsletter* containing the reports, Health Canada said that changes had been made to the Prepulsid's official drug profile, including updated prescribing information.

On January 24, 2000, the FDA sent out another letter advising patients to have an electrocardiogram before taking Prepulsid. The administration also said the drug should *not be prescribed to patients with eating disorders.*

A warning letter was sent to Canadian doctors on February 25, 2000, at which time Health Canada decided to review the drug more thoroughly. Prepulsid was withdrawn from the U.S. market on March 23, 2000, and from the Canadian market on May 31, 2000. As of August 7, 2000, the drug was no longer available in Canada. At the time of withdrawal, Health Canada said that it had received 44 reports of potential heart rhythm abnormalities, including 10 deaths associated with the drug. In the United States, Prepulsid had been associated with 341 serious adverse reactions and at least 80 deaths.

In April 2000, a few weeks after Vanessa's death, Terence obtained a copy of the *U.S. Prepulsid Medication Guide*, the information sheet given to American patients with their pills. Key sections included:

What is the Most Important Information I Should Know About Prepulsid (cisapride)?

- PREPULSID may cause serious irregular heartbeats that may cause death.
- If you feel faint, become dizzy or have irregular heartbeats while using PREPULSID, stop taking PREPULSID and get medical help right away.
- Also, you should not take PREPULSID if you have any of these conditions [four of the nine conditions follow]
    1. low levels of potassium, calcium or magnesium
    2. an eating disorder (such as bulimia and anorexia)
    3. your body has suddenly lost a lot of water
    4. persistent vomiting

- The safety and effectiveness of PREPULSID in children younger than 16 years has not been demonstrated for any use. Serious adverse events, including death, have been reported in infants and children while being treated with PREPULSID, although there is no clear evidence that PREPULSID caused them.

Vanessa displayed all four of these conditions. As a bulimic, she vomited, which can lead to dehydration and the loss of chemicals such as potassium, calcium and magnesium. Imbalance of these chemicals affects the functioning of heart muscle and the nervous system.

At the time patients in the United States were being warned that Prepulsid could cause irregular heartbeats, possibly with fatal outcomes, Canadians were being told the drug had few or no side effects. Why did Canadians not see this up-front, clearly worded warning about the adverse reactions to Prepulsid? Where was Health Canada?

A coroner's inquest that began exactly one year after Vanessa's death found the cause of death to be acute hypoxic/ischemic encephalopathy (lack of oxygen to the brain) due to arrhythmia followed by cardiac arrest resulting from the effects of bulimia nervosa in conjunction with cisapride (Prepulsid) toxicity and possibly an unknown co-factor such as congenital cardiac defect. This multi-faceted cause allowed the drug company, Vanessa's doctors and Health Canada to exempt themselves from any blame or responsibility. The purpose of an inquest is to find fact, not to lay blame.

Facts to emerge during the inquest that concluded on April 24, 2001, revealed that prescription drugs, which can be highly beneficial, even life-saving, are one of Canada's most serious and under-reported causes of health problems.

"The federal government should review why the system is failing to protect Canadians against dangerous drugs," Terence told the coroner's jury as part of his own long list of recommendations. Among his other recommendations were to advise patients in clear language of all risks and benefits associated with a drug; make it mandatory for drug companies, doctors and pharmacists to immediately report any adverse drug reactions to Health Canada; and implement stiff fines for drug companies and sales representatives that withhold important drug safety information.

At the top of the jury's 59 recommendations was establishing a national body to examine how critical drug safety information is delivered to Canadians. Relevant recommendations were directed to the pharmaceutical industry, the Ontario College of Physicians and Surgeons, Ontario College of Pharmacists, Ontario College of Family Physicians, Ontario Medical Schools, Ontario College of Nurses, Ontario Ministry of Health, Coroner's Office of Ontario and Health Canada. In November 2010, Young said that of the 16 key recommendations for Health Canada, only a few had been implemented, and they were "easy stuff" such as developing a website and setting up a toll-free number for general inquiries regarding drug information for the general public.

In a December 21, 2006, report, Jenny Manzer of the *Ottawa Citizen* newspaper wrote, "There are many facets of our drug safety system that might surprise Canadians, particularly how closely Health Canada works with the drug industry." Two years earlier, the Canadian Association of Journalists selected Health Canada for the Code of Silence Award for its repeated refusals to make the database that contains drug side effects available to journalists and researchers. Subsequently, the database was made public.

At the conclusion of the inquest, Gary Will, the lawyer representing the Young family, told the *National Post* newspaper, as reported by Anne Marie Owens on April 25, 2001, that he was not surprised when Janssen's spokeswoman walked away from reporters when asked if the company accepted any responsibility for the death: "This company spent four weeks at the inquest trying to blame Vanessa Young and trying to blame the Young family. They didn't take responsibility for their actions." He also said that a larger federal inquiry is necessary to uncover what he called the Prepulsid scandal and to answer important questions such as, "Why did Janssen continue marketing this drug when they knew people were dying? Why are they marketing this drug to 100 countries around the world today?"

In July 2001, Terence initiated a $100 million class-action lawsuit against Health Canada and Janssen-Ortho Corporation for allegedly failing to notify patients about the potentially harmful side effects of Prepulsid. From its approval in 1990 until 2001, Prepulsid was prescribed as a "heartburn drug" to approximately a million Canadians. In April 2001, a man in Sault Ste. Marie, Ontario, filed a $600 million class-action motion. The man allegedly had two heart attacks after taking the drug. In the United States, there were more than 500 individual and class-action lawsuits against the pharmaceutical company and doctors before the courts in 2001 regarding the side effects of Prepulsid.

In January 2007, a judge ruled that the class-action suit initiated by Terence could move toward trial. The decision to certify the case followed years of legal wrangling. The drug company appealed the certification, but lost in May 2007. They appealed the appeal decision and again lost. Although pleased with the decision, supporters of the suit were concerned that it had taken six years to get the case to this stage. A similar case in the United States was settled in 2004 with a payout of up to US$90 million to 16,000 Prepulsid users.

While the class-action suit was moving toward certification, Terence and his family pursued a separate individual lawsuit, which was settled in February 2006. Although wanting a public trial to expose alleged failures, Terence was unwilling to risk having to pay the legal costs of the defendants if he lost. The thought of losing the family home was too much to contemplate on top of all his family had suffered. "There is no balance of power between powerless individuals and huge international corporations as there is in the U.S.," he wrote.

In 2002, Terence founded the organization Drug Safety Canada (DSC), which is dedicated to reducing the number of patient deaths and serious adverse reactions by improving prescription drug safety. Looking to the future, DSC wants a new perspective on health care, one in which "pharmaceuticals do not dominate medicine and are prescribed only when they will be truly safe for patients. This would reduce patient deaths in North America by as much as 140,000 a year and reduce serious injuries by over 1,000,000 per year."

We believe that prescribing a drug safely should include the doctor's full medical understanding of two things:

- the true risks of the drug for each patient, taking into consideration not just their symptoms, but their condition, age, sex and all other drugs and natural health products they are taking, along with foods they are consuming.
- the proven efficacy of the drug for that patient, using the best available objective evidence, based on reports of adverse reaction injuries and deaths in every country where the drug is marketed.

Patients should provide informed consent for each prescription after hearing the true potential risks along with the proven potential benefits of any therapy and after receiving professional advice on possible alternatives to prescription drug therapy, such as changes in work, diet, exercise and sleep habits, and other safer therapies that are clinically proven to benefit patients.

DSC's website also provides information regarding prescription drugs by citing studies from recognized medical, scientific and government sources.

Terence is a stalwart supporter of other families whose children and other members have died under circumstances in which prescription drugs may have played a role. "Sara Carlin hanged herself," an upset Hart Young told his family after taking a phone call at 9 p.m. on May 7, 2007. Sara, 18, belonged to Hart's group of friends and had been at the Young house a few weeks earlier.

Terence's first thought was about the family and what they must be feeling. His second thought was suspicion. A beautiful, vibrant girl, Sara had been a high achiever at school until early 2006 when she had been prescribed the SSRI antidepressant Paxil, and her behaviour began to change. She quit sports and her part-time job, suffered from insomnia and became involved with recreational drugs and alcohol. No one had told Sara or her family that Health Canada had already issued two warning letters to health-care professionals about Paxil and suicide. The second letter in particular warned about the risk of self-harm and behavioural and emotional changes, including agitation, hostility, depersonalization and several symptoms that could manifest as an almost indescribable sense of terror and doom. "Sara had apparently hung herself in the basement of her home some time on Saturday night. Her father found her fully suspended at 4:30 p.m. on Sunday. I could only imagine his horror," Terence wrote.

An inquest into Sara's death was held in summer 2010. Terence's testimony at the inquest was described by David Lea in a June 18, 2010, article in the *Oakville Beaver* newspaper as showing no mercy for Health Canada, GlaxoSmithKline (manufacturer of Paxil) and others for not doing enough to protect Canadians from the dangers of prescription drugs. During the two-week-long inquest, some experts argued there was no evidence that Paxil caused Sara's suicide, while the Carlin family, their lawyer and others maintained she became increasingly depressed after starting to take Paxil in February 2006.

The inquest resulted in 16 recommendations, including a call for the federal government to create an arm's-length body called the Drug Safety Board to investigate the side effects of prescription drugs and issue warnings to the public, doctors and hospitals. This recommendation came after Terence told the inquest that Health Canada's use of trials partly funded by pharmaceutical companies to decide which drugs to put on the market creates a bias. He also recommended that drug companies be required to publish the results of all their clinical trials, not just the favourable ones, and that patients should be made aware if the drug they are taking has a history of adverse reactions in other countries. In addition, health-care professionals should be required to report all suspected adverse drug reactions to Health Canada within 48 hours of the reaction taking place.

At the time of the inquest, Terence, who had been elected Member of Provincial Parliament representing Oakville, Ontario, two years earlier, had a private member's motion before the Legislative Assembly. Bill M-355 states: "That, in the opinion of the House, the government should create an arm's-length Independent Drug Agency similar to the Transportation Safety Board and Canadian Nuclear Safety Commission, to be responsible for making and keeping Canadians safe when using prescription drugs and over-the-counter drugs, and for reducing injuries and deaths caused by or related to their use." The proposed agency would have the power to order (not negotiate) unsafe drugs off the market, and the power to distribute clearly worded warnings to doctors and patients for all approved drugs. At the Carlin inquest, Terence said it would be some time before the motion would be discussed. The situation remained the same two years later.

When Terence ran for federal office in 2008, he promised to be an additional voice in Ottawa for improved regulations, especially about the need for effective safety warnings given to patients with their pre-scriptions. He also promised to work toward ending the inappropriate partnerships between large pharmaceutical companies and doctors and regulators. On January 24, 2011, Terence told CTV News: "Nothing significant has changed since Vanessa died. There are dangerous drugs on the market right now, because regulators still aren't issuing proper safety warnings. Twenty-two prescription drugs that Health Canada and the pharmaceutical industry told us were safe have been taken off the market since 1977 for injuring and killing patients."

Always concerned about health issues, especially those related to children, Terence supported the government's regulations announced in January 2011 to restrict the use of six phthalates, chemicals that may case adverse health effects in children and infants, in toys and childcare items. Terence was re-elected as MPP for Oakville in the May 2011.

On March 26, 2009, Terence made a presentation to the Ontario Legislative Assembly Standing Committee on Justice Policy, which was considering changes to the Coroner's Act. Terence was joined by Neil Carlin, Sara's father, and Maryanne Murray, whose 22-year-old daughter, Martha, died in September 2002 after being given lithium when it was contraindicated. All three parents wanted the addition of a new category in the classification of deaths for those deaths caused by administration of drugs. The existing categories are natural, acci-dental, homicide, suicide and undetermined. Terence explained to the committee the rationale for proposing the new category: "Our chief concern is that deaths caused by prescription drugs are almost always classified under the act as 'natural.' You read that right. According to the Ontario Coroner's Act deaths caused by an adverse reaction to a drugs are classified as 'natural.' The only way to help reduce drug deaths is to identify the problem, not cover it up. We are calling for a new fifth category in the act." The parents' proposal was not adopted.

Terence's well-researched book, *Death by Prescription*, was released in April 2009. At the book's launch, Terence spoke about how pharmaceuticals came to dominate medical care, citing that more is spent on drugs ($24 billion in 2005 in prescription and over-the-counter sales of drugs) than on doctors ($18 billion). In the meantime, more than 100,000 Canadians and more than two million people in the U.S. are seriously injured each year.

Death by Prescription contains many of Terence's thought-provoking insights:

> I had always thought risk management referred to the risk to the patients. I remembered what Alex Demerse had told me. "From their [the pharmaceutical companies] view, it's better to keep selling it if the lawsuits are minimal — especially in Canada. It's just the cost of doing business." If they start losing in court, he'd said, their insurance will cover most of the costs. So that was risk management. It wasn't the risk to patients they were worried about. It was risk to the corporation! Risk management is a practice that puts human life on the same continuum as money. Money versus lives. Lives versus money [. . .]
>
> In 2003 a leading expert on prescription drugs made an astonishing statement at a scientific meeting in London, England. Dr. Allen Roses, vice-president of genetics for GlaxoSmith Kline (GSK), the world's second-largest drug company, reported, "The vast majority of drugs — more than 90 percent — only work in 30 or 50 percent of people." GSK marketed the blockbusters Advair, Avandia, Paxil, Zophran, Wellbutrin and Augmentin . . . Prescription drug sales hit the $600 billion mark worldwide in 2006. Dr. Roses was saying indirectly that perhaps $200 billion a year spent worldwide on prescription drugs is really wasted.

And since all drugs cause adverse reactions, millions of patients are put at risk daily for no good reason [. . .]

The Canadian Pharmacists' Association says that the cost of underuse, misuse, and overuse of prescription drugs could range between $2 billion and $9 billion a year. How much healthier would Canadians be if we invested that money in preventative health care, such as regular checkups, physical activity, stress management, diet education, tobacco intervention, and tests like pap smears and colonoscopies? . . .

Gloria and I had always taught our children they were incredibly lucky to live in Canada. I recalled a happy time — the first time we listened to Vanessa and her classmates sing "O Canada" — her grade one concert at Abbey Lane School. "We stand on guard for thee," the children sang. But shouldn't loyalty work both ways? Wasn't there an unspoken promise for the government to stand on guard for Vanessa? The government and Health Canada have broken faith with the rest of us. And Vanessa paid the ultimate price.

Terence wrote his book to save lives and to fulfill an oath he had made the day after Vanessa died — to find out why and how she died. In the book's epilogue, he wrote:

Who killed Vanessa? When it was all said and done, I think the ultimate enemy was self-interest. Professional people in positions of trust neglected to do what they knew they should have. Others concerned about their jobs and careers turned a blind eye to dangers to which they would never have exposed their own families. They turned off their sense of right and wrong when they went to work each day.

But the people who casually manipulated the self-interest of others, and acted to delay and undermine effective warnings that would have saved Vanessa's life deserve special recognition.

Forever Changed

It wasn't the slip of the surgeon's scalpel or almost dying from the consequences or the prolonged painful recovery that made Rhonda Nixon a health-care advocate; it was the deception, consistent denial of wrongdoing and the frustration of trying to work with the health authority. During a procedure to discover and correct the cause of complications following surgery to remove her gallbladder, Rhonda's duodenum (the upper portion of her small bowel) and common bile duct were perforated. In her search for answers about what had happened and why communications with her health-care providers and the health authority were so poor, Rhonda found almost no relevant information available in Canada.

The turning point came when she connected with American leaders in the field of patient safety. Four years after the surgery, Rhonda and her husband organized "The Empowered Patient Conference: Including the Patient in Patient Safety," held in Nanaimo, BC, on November 7, 2009, to highlight Canadian Patient Safety Week. The meeting provided participants with the type of information Rhonda wished she'd had during her ordeal. Rhonda subsequently founded the society Empowered Patient Canada, with the intent of helping to prevent errors in the Canadian health-care system by providing education and information to the public. Rhonda continues to provide information and support to a wide spectrum of people faced with navigating the health-care system.

Surgery

On May 3, 2005, Rhonda Nixon, 39, underwent laparoscopic surgery to remove her gallbladder following an episode of acute pancreatitis several months earlier. The surgeon told Rhonda he had not found any gallstones. Rhonda went home the next day anticipating an uneventful recovery. In the second week after surgery, Rhonda returned to work as a loans officer at a local financial institution. On the morning of June 1, she collapsed in her kitchen from a sudden squeezing spasm that took her breath away. The spasm subsided in a few minutes. Rhonda went to work the next day. The morning of June 3, another spasm incapacitated her at work and she was taken by ambulance to the general hospital where her gallbladder had been removed.

The ER physician ordered blood tests. He told Rhonda the results indicated that the common bile duct might be blocked and she would probably need a procedure called an endoscopic retrograde cholangio-pancreatogram (ERCP). This procedure combines the use of a flexible lighted scope (endoscope) with x-ray pictures to examine the ducts that drain the liver, gallbladder and pancreas. Rhonda was released the next day with instructions to return if she had another attack.

On the evening of June 6, she experienced an intense burning pain down her right side and noticed a small bulge in her right flank. "I have to go back," she told her husband, Gord, a Royal Canadian Mounted Police officer. At the hospital, Rhonda spoke to two surgeons who thought it best that the ERCP be done by the surgeon, Dr. S., who had removed her gallbladder. "He knows your ducts better than anyone else," she was told. Rhonda went home on June 8 to await the ERCP procedure that was scheduled for June 21. "I never believed the hospital would be unsafe or I would need someone with me," she said.

In addition to the ERCP, Dr. S. performed a sphincterotomy, a cutting of the muscle that lies at the juncture of the intestine with both the bile and pancreatic ducts. "Never did I expect them to do anything while they were in there," said Rhonda. Later, in the post-anesthetic recovery room, Rhonda remembers a nurse with a clipboard stopping at the foot of her bed and exclaiming, "Oh, my God, she didn't sign the consent form."

A few minutes later, Dr. S. came to see Rhonda, who was experiencing considerable pain in the groin area when she moved her right leg. He leaned close and whispered to Rhonda that he would be keeping her overnight for observation, because he may have nicked her bowel. He asked her repeatedly if she understood and if she would remember what he had said. Irritated at his insistence, Rhonda sat up and said, "I'm one of the sharpest tacks in the box. I will not forget." When Dr. S. called Gord to say he was keeping Rhonda in overnight, he said that he may have nicked her bowel. Dr. S. later denied that these conversations ever occurred.

Two days after the surgery, Gord arrived at the hospital to take Rhonda home, only to be met by a nurse who told him how glad they were he was there. His wife had taken an unexpected turn for the worse and was being rushed to the ICU. The "unexpected turn" had occurred much earlier, but no one had called Gord. Rhonda recalls the worst month of her life:

> I was severely ill and kept in ICU for 10 days. I experienced many complications/adverse events which included but were not limited to: bile duct perforation, sepsis, peritonitis, respiratory failure as indicated by early ARDS [acute respiratory distress syndrome], perforation and collapse of both lungs caused by incorrect insertion of a pigtail catheter chest tube, bilateral pleural effusions, aspiration pneumonia due to inhalation of GI contents and collection of large amounts of fluid in my abdomen that required several months of drainage. I was also MRSA+.
>
> The pain was intense.
>
> I tried very hard to keep aware of what was going on around me, but as my condition worsened I overheard that I might end up being put on a ventilator. If this happened, I knew I would be unable to speak and thought I might die. I asked Gord to write down my instructions for paying our bills and to get the power of attorney document from our safety deposit box. I also asked Gord to ask my father to come, because I wanted to see him before I died and he could help look after our boys.

I spent 10 days in ICU and 30 days altogether in the hospital. I was in isolation the whole time due to being MRSA+. While in hospital, I suffered medication errors and observed poor sanitation practices. Gord and I kept asking for information about my condition, but received little information. Everyone we asked would refer us to someone else. We would receive responses such as "it's hard to say" or "I don't know." We were going in circles.

Finally, I requested to leave the hospital. I knew I had to get home. The longer I stayed the worse I became. If I was going to die, it would be at home. Gord spoke to Dr. S., who said I was in no shape to go home. Gord then took him for a walk and when they returned, Dr. S. said he'd try to get me home in four days.

Recovery, Realization and Frustration

Incredibly weak, Rhonda came home on July 20 to face a long and difficult recovery. She required a drain to remove fluid from her abdomen and visits from a home-care nurse twice a day for five months. Among other symptoms, she suffered intense epigastric spasms which continued intermittently for two years. Gord took seven weeks off work to care for Rhonda, and her father moved into their home for two months to assist. Rhonda did not return to work for almost a year. Rhonda's injuries and illness had a profound effect on those around her, especially her two sons, who were 14 and 11 years old at the time. Her oldest son subsequently told the health authority's director of risk management, "We want you to know that you have taken our mother from us. She is not the same person she once was."

Several weeks after she returned home, the home-care nurse told Rhonda that she was a walking miracle. The comment increased Gord and Rhonda's curiosity about exactly what had happened. In spite of repeated attempts to get information from both Dr. S. and Rhonda's general practitioner, Dr. G., they did not learn anything of substance. They were consistently told that the problem was complications of post-ERCP pancreatitis. Gord asked the surgeon three times, twice in the ICU and once on the phone, if there had been a perforation.

The surgeon said there hadn't been a perforation and denied ever telling Rhonda that he may have nicked her bowel during the ERCP. Rhonda recalls:

> Around Labour Day [2005], it struck me that I had been deceived. A friend who is a registered nurse had previously said she hoped I was keeping a journal. At the time I didn't understand why I would need to keep a written record of events. When I realized that there might be something going on that I didn't know about, I wrote down everything that had happened and kept a journal from then on.
>
> At a follow-up office visit in late November, my surgeon unintentionally revealed to me that he had made a small perforation in my common bile duct during the ERCP/sphincterotomy performed in June. I had been led to believe that I was suffering these severe complications as a result of post-ERCP pancreatitis.
>
> The truth was withheld from my family and me for five months. Without this critical information, my health could have been further jeopardized should I have travelled outside the Vancouver Island Health Authority jurisdiction where doctors would not have had ready access to my medical records. It has since become apparent to me that during my 10-day stay in the ICU there was atelectasis [partial or complete collapse of a lung] and duodenal damage, and my life was indeed in danger. Neither my husband nor I were informed of the severity of my condition.
>
> Two days later during another office visit to my surgeon, I confronted him about the undisclosed perforation. He was upset and apologetic. I requested a second opinion. In January 2006, I received a second opinion from a specialist who confirmed that I had experienced a duodenal leak. He informed me that my six months of complications were a direct result of a perforation, not of pancreatitis as I had been consistently told.

In March 2006, Rhonda returned to work and requested all her medical records from the health authority. She specifically asked for "all medical reports and investigations, notes, consent releases and any other documents related to my care not specifically mentioned in this request." She was astounded to receive only an inch-thick stack of records, because she had seen doctors and nurses consulting two large binders while in hospital. She insisted on receiving her complete records from the authority. They arrived in late April. That was when Rhonda realized that her condition while in ICU was nearly fatal and that neither she nor Gord were told the truth despite their repeated requests for information.

Rhonda again felt deceived, because she learned from CT scan reports in her medical records that a perforation or perforations had occurred. The reports were available to both Dr. S. and Dr. G., yet both doctors denied knowledge of a perforation. The specific site(s) of the perforation(s), common bile duct, duodenum or both, are not identified in the reports. Immediately following the ERCP, Dr. S. told Rhonda he had nicked her bowel and this was later confirmed by a specialist's opinion. Yet in the late November office visit, he told Rhonda there had been a perforation of the common bile duct. The common bile duct is in close proximity to the duodenum.

Rhonda believes that when Dr. S. learned she had not signed the consent form, he arranged to have it included in the hospital admitting forms that she was asked to sign after the procedure while recovering from sedation. Rhonda signed the forms. She also discovered mistakes in her medical records about which surgeon had performed the surgery and the identity of the attending nurses. Subsequently, corrections to the records were appended. (Medical records are considered legal documents and cannot be altered. However, documents correcting earlier statements or opinions can be added.)

In Rhonda's words:

> Dr. S. and Dr. G. went to great lengths not to disclose that any perforation(s) had occurred. In my opinion, meaningful communication between myself and my caregivers was sabotaged once they realized the consent form had not been signed and I would ultimately survive with long-term complications.
>
> I felt betrayed by two doctors whom I trusted to put my care above their own reputations. It's bad enough that I almost died as a result

of the procedure performed, but the ongoing emotional and physical trauma that I have been left with has been devastating. I accept that possible complications come with all surgical procedures; however, I will never accept that physicians have a right to misinform, lie and cover up medical errors such that their patients' rights and safety are placed at risk.

The following weeks, months and years brought a long series of frustrations to the Nixons, especially considering their desire to work with medical professionals and the health authority. What the Nixons thought would be a simple trail to the truth in order to help others became a tangled web. Rhonda came to the conclusion that authorities often had good intentions, but appeared to lack adequate investigative skills and knowledge about consent, disclosure and apology policies.

Throughout the years, the Nixons were crystal clear that their objective was to improve the health-care system by working with it, not against it. In her letter of April 2007 to the complaints department of the College of Physicians and Surgeons of British Columbia, Rhonda wrote:

In closing, I would like to point out that mistakes happen, but we are measured by how we deal with those mistakes. I have consciously dismissed litigation in favour of this process [contacting the College] as I believe we all have a great deal to learn from my misfortune.

Ultimately I believe that both my surgeon and general practitioner are working within a flawed system where medical professionals fear and rarely admit their mistakes due to medical-legal consequences. This complaint is an effort to address this flaw. If I had been promptly and fully informed and these physicians had been up front and honest immediately, I would still be working with them today on my ongoing physical and emotional issues.

The College eventually replied that nothing in the doctors' practice with regard to Rhonda's complaints warranted remediation or discipline. However, the complaints committee was of the opinion that the discharge summary, dictated months later, was lacking relevant details and stated that Dr. S. would be advised of this.

In response to her request to obtain the health authority's consent policy, Rhonda received a phone call from the director of risk management. She didn't know the reason for his call, but her concern increased when he said he'd personally read all of her charts and offered to meet with the Nixons in their home.

The risk manager arrived on April 19, 2007, thinking he was going to talk about informed consent. Instead, Rhonda presented him with a banker's box filled with her medical records related to the June 2005 surgical error and the Nixons' subsequent investigation of seven specific complaints and 34 additional concerns. The manager asked several times who had compiled and organized the information for them. Gord, an experienced police officer, repeatedly answered that Rhonda and he had done it themselves. "I used the technique police call the tip system, which was employed in complex police investigations prior to implementation of computer-based systems. It is a simple process which assigns a separate file for every piece of information received and each respective complaint so that all information is assessed, cross-referenced and collated for ease of understanding and processing. (See Investigative Tip System at page 215 for details.) Gord suspects that no one in health care had seen the technique before and that no one had any training in investigative techniques.

During the five-hour meeting with the risk manager, the Nixons emphasized that they had no intention of suing the health authority, but only wanted to use Rhonda's experience as a learning tool for health-care providers and the health authority on how to handle disclosure of adverse events and apologies.

At the top of their seven complaints were failure to disclose that a perforation had occurred, failure to obtain lawful consent prior to the ERCP/sphincterotomy, and withholding information by failure to disclose the surgical error. Other complaints included Rhonda's general practitioner's failure to read the surgical reports and provide appropriate follow-up care, and an apparent attempt to hide perforation-related injuries. Inadequate and incorrect documentation were also concerns.

After months of investigation, the risk manager reported that "not one thing had been found" and "no evidence of 'negligence' could be found." But Rhonda had never alleged or even mentioned negligence. "They spent all those resources investigating something I never complained about," she said. Gord and Rhonda asked for complaint guidelines, a root cause analysis study and consent policy guidelines, never mentioning negligence. They tried to reach the CEO of the health authority, without success. The Nixons met with senior executives of the health authority only to leave frustrated, because the executives were not prepared for the meeting and did not understand Rhonda's objective.

A later report from the health authority stated that there was a lack of timely and coordinated response to Rhonda's concerns and that the transfer of documentation and communication between programs was inadequate to maintain continuity of care. Further, the medical staff rules and regulations did not support completion of health records in a timely way. The absence of documentation of the time when consent for the ERCP was obtained and the lack of documentation of conversations between Rhonda and her physicians were also points of concern. The report recommended that a formal apology be extended to Rhonda and her family on behalf of all her care providers for the long and difficult episode of care.

On November 29, 2007, the *Nanaimo Daily News* ran a feature article, "Routine Surgery Causes Injury: A Parksville Woman Demanded Answers, and Was Shocked at What She Found." A week later, Howard Waldner, president and CEO of the health authority, apologized to Rhonda and her family in a letter to the paper's editor. Rhonda was not impressed. "I had been sent home to die and he apologizes indirectly through a letter to the editor. His letter was written for the public, not me," she said.

In his letter, Waldner wrote that the health authority was implementing a number of initiatives to improve communication and procedures including restructuring of the complaint, concern and care follow-up process. As well, staff were being provided with education on disclosure of information to patients and consent procedures. A quality and patient safety advisory committee was being established to provide patient input into the health authority's patient safety activities.

The Nixons had further communications and meetings with various health executives. Prior to one meeting, they sent letters to the executive office. The letters outlined some of their ongoing concerns and were addressed to each board member. Apparently, the letters were intercepted in the office because the board members never received them. The executive in charge of the office appeared stunned as police officer Gord told the board that interception of lawful delivery of mail was a criminal offence.

Connecting

Rhonda, with Gord's assistance, organized "The Empowered Patient Conference: Including the Patient in Patient Safety," held in Nanaimo, BC, on November 7, 2009, to highlight Canadian Patient Safety Week. The focus was on creating a greater awareness of patient safety issues and providing participants with the information and knowledge needed to help them become better advocates. By all measures, the conference was a resounding success. With little advance publicity, over 175 people from across Canada and several from the United States came to hear well-recognized authorities speak on how to become an informed patient and how to deal with unanticipated outcomes.

In her introductory comments, Rhonda told those in attendance about her own search for information, the people who helped her and how the conference came about.

> As I recovered, my husband and I tried to find out what had caused the complications and what treatments, if any, might help in my recovery. What we had been told occurred did not make sense given the information we were gathering from outside the hospital. I began to wonder

how it was that I knew so little about my condition. I did not understand the inadequate communication we were experiencing with my health-care providers. The more questions we asked the more distant my health-care providers became. To find answers, I started searching the internet.

I soon realized that there was little information in Canada for a patient who had experienced a medically induced trauma — often referred to as an "adverse event" or "iatrogenic injury." I also learned that it was common for a patient who had experienced a medically induced trauma to be treated as a pariah. My spirit was breaking. I realized that if my condition had been caused by cancer or another illness there would be information, resources and support available. Someone would have been there for me.

And so I wondered: How often do these adverse events occur? Why were my questions going unanswered? What information and resources are available for the patient and family when an adverse event occurs? I then began thinking about the health-care providers: What does a health-care professional experience when they are involved in or cause an adverse event? And finally I began asking something we all should be asking: What process does the institution/organization follow after a medical error/adverse event? What is the reporting and disclosure process following such an event?

Through my inquiries, I learned about people like Dr. John Banja, a professor of ethics at Emory University in Atlanta, Georgia, who referred me to a patient advocate named Ilene Corina, founder and president of PULSE in New York. I called Ilene, who asked for my email address and told me that within a few hours the leaders in the field of patient safety would arrive in my inbox. The emails arrived just as she said they would. I was overwhelmed. The network consists of grassroots advocates, survivors and medical providers all working to improve the health-care system. Most were from the United States. While the American health-care system is different from ours, the issues surrounding patient safety are the same.

One of the leaders who arrived in my inbox was Helen Haskell, founder and president of Mothers Against Medical Errors. Helen and I corresponded and she recently introduced me to Dr. Julia Hallisy, author of *The Empowered Patient.* I had already started thinking about holding a conference on Patient Safety when last May my husband and I attended Dr. Hallisy's Empowered Patient Healthcare Conference in San Francisco. It was a great experience and I knew a similar conference would be of benefit here in Canada. Since then, Helen and Julia have co-founded and launched the Empowered Patient Coalition. Of all the information I have come across, it has been their work which resonates most with me.

Over the past four years, as word got out about my experience and interest in patient safety, people who had experienced similar situations began to contact me for information. They contacted me both at home and work, and I was happy to share the information that I had acquired. I am not an expert, so I tried to engage my local health authority in an effort to have my case used as a learning tool for others. This effort did not work, so I considered alternatives. I wondered what the response would be if I organized an event to bring that information directly to the people most interested in patient safety.

This event started out small. I asked Helen and Julia if they would come to Nanaimo. Their response was positive. They were equally as positive when I mentioned names of the diverse group of speakers you will hear today.

Every patient advocate that I've talked to says the same thing; they are forever changed. They wish no other family to endure the same preventable nightmare they experienced. These advocates share their stories so that you may learn and become an active partner in your own health care. We are all vulnerable to error. Health-care error occurs at the best facilities even with the finest doctors and nurses. In my own experience these health-care professionals want nothing but the best for their clients, and when an unanticipated event occurs, it can be as devastating for them as it is for the patient and family. Health-care professionals never intend to harm. How they and their institutions react will make all the difference in how the patient and family overcome the adverse event.

Patients and their families are entitled to full disclosure so that they may make informed decisions about their immediate, ongoing and future care. There must be support and resources available for the patient, family and caregiver as soon as the health-care professionals realize that an error has occurred. This must be mandated by government and there must be consequences for those who fail to disclose such errors.

Patients must also become more "empowered" and share in the responsibility to make informed choices about their own health care. Taking better care of ourselves will lead to reduced health-care costs at a time when these costs are skyrocketing. By doing this, we not only help ourselves, but we also help our community and employers in these difficult economic times. We cannot afford to be passive bystanders any longer. We need to have *high* expectations of ourselves and we need to have *high* expectations of our health-care providers. It is time for all of us to become "empowered patients."

In 2010, Rhonda founded the Empowered Patient Canada (EPC) Society, for which she serves as president. The purposes of the society were to provide education and information to increase understanding of patient safety and error prevention in the Canadian health-care system. As a result of the conference and the society, Rhonda participated in a number of studies, workshops and round-table discussion groups. Local media outlets frequently contacted her for interviews on various aspects of patient safety. People affected by errors continue to ask Rhonda for information and advice. Excerpts from recent emails follow:

> *From a care aide who was off work and could not get help and with whom Rhonda had extensive correspondence:* I want to thank you so much for your time and support. I felt so much better after our talk. I'd expressed my feelings to people before, but it's not the same when they don't really "get it" or have been there. Your links are great too. Keep them coming!

> *From a woman responding to the EPC website:* I know we've not yet had the opportunity to speak/meet but I was hoping you could help me. I have a friend whose sister died suddenly a few weeks ago and

the family feels mistakes were made. With your permission, I'd like to give her your contact information. Possibly my friend could connect with you via Facebook and hopefully by sharing your story and your experiences, you might be able to help her family in some way, shape or form.

In the years since her surgery, Rhonda has made significant contributions to the information available to Canadians affected by medical errors. In addition, she provides that all-important aspect of the person who has been there. The long-term effects of advocacy work such as Rhonda's are impossible to measure; however, one known result is this book. Susan McIver's interest in medical errors was rekindled when Rhonda asked her to join the board of EPC nine years after the publication of her first book, *Medical Nightmares: The Human Face of Errors*.

Hear My Voice

A retired teacher full of life, Esther Winckler, 77, entered hospital for elective hip replacement surgery on February 20, 2000. Contraindicated by her medical history and without any documentation of her consent, she was given a general anesthetic. Postoperative congestive heart failure was not recognized and not treated. She fell twice and sustained severe head injuries that were not thoroughly investigated. No one noticed that she did not have a bowel movement in her 15-day hospitalization. Lack of oxygen in her system caused Esther to suffer delirium, which was managed by restraining her in a wheelchair with a leather belt strapped around her painfully distended abdomen. The coroner's report released over two years after Esther's death revealed disturbing deficiencies in 10 areas of care she had received at an acute care general hospital. Esther died from lack of oxygen and destruction of tissue in her brain and bowel as a result of critically low oxygen and blood pressure levels over a prolonged period.

Esther's family — husband Lawrence, daughter Catherine and son Ron — wanted to know why things had gone so wrong. Although they first encountered a wall of silence, they persevered in their determination to work with, not against, the health-care system. Catherine established a website called Esther's Voice (EsthersVoice.com) which, combined with the coroner's report and a series of prominent articles in the Vancouver Sun newspaper, tore down the wall of silence. Esther's voice continues to improve the care and save the lives of countless patients, especially the elderly, in Canada and elsewhere thanks in large part to a few dedicated BC nurses and also to health authority officials who listened. Catherine continues to receive calls and emails from across Canada and overseas from nurses, other health-care professionals and families.

Catherine and her family's leadership have yielded results beyond anything they could have imagined.

Preoperative Assessment to Death

In early 2000, Esther Winckler, 77, agreed to have elective hip replacement surgery at a general hospital in British Columbia. She anticipated that once free of the pain from her osteoarthritic hip she would be able to resume travelling. Regardless of the ongoing pain, Esther, who was often described as "feisty," gardened, cooked and managed the home she shared with her husband, Lawrence, a retired businessman. As a teacher in a Vancouver high school, Esther had pioneered a home economics course for immigrants and First Nations students who were seeking jobs in hospitals and private homes. In retirement, she remained actively engaged in the world around her.

Esther's previous surgeries included removal of her right lung in 1986 because of cancer. She also had asthma, chronic obstructive lung disease and hypertension (high blood pressure). In 1994, during back surgery performed under a general anesthetic, she had a life-threatening experience. The surgery, scheduled as a double decompression at two levels of her spine, was aborted after the first decompression, because Esther's blood pressure and oxygen saturation dropped to dangerous levels. The following year, Esther fractured her right hip, which healed without incident.

On February 2, 2000, Esther underwent a preoperative assessment at the hospital. The assessment included blood work, physical assessment, x-rays of the left hip and chest and an anesthesia questionnaire. The anesthetist, Dr. A., concluded that, in view of Esther's medical history, she should have a spinal anesthetic. Dr. A. documented that he had discussed this with Esther and she agreed. In fact, not only did she agree, but according to her daughter, Catherine, consenting to surgery was conditional upon having a spinal anesthetic.

On February 20, 2000, Esther was admitted to the hospital and underwent various tests to assess respiratory function. All test results were within normal ranges. In the evening, a preoperative anesthetic assessment was performed by a different anesthetist than the one who had conducted the first assessment 18 days earlier. This anesthetist, Dr. B., would be administering the anesthetic during surgery. He classified Esther as having severe systemic disease. She had asthma, chronic obstructive pulmonary disease and only one lung. This limited her activity, but did not cause incapacitation. There is no documentation in Esther's medical records regarding a discussion about the type of anesthetic to be used.

Later that evening, Catherine found a message on her phone recorder from Esther saying that she was very upset, because Dr. B. had told her she would undergo general anesthesia the following morning. Catherine was also concerned. She was unable to reach Esther's general practitioner or surgeon before the surgery, which was slated for early in the morning.

On the morning of February 21, 2000, the anesthetist, Dr. B., administered epidural (not to be confused with a spinal anesthetic) and general anesthetics, and the orthopedic surgeon performed a total left hip replacement. Esther remained in stable condition throughout surgery, which was completed at 10:15 a.m. During the procedure, Esther received 2750 cc of fluid and excreted only 800 cc, leaving a positive fluid balance of approximately 2000 cc.

Upon her arrival in the post-anaesthetic care unit (PACU), Esther's blood pressure was within the normal range, but quickly dropped until it reached 97/58 half an hour later. Her oxygen saturation was 96 percent, within the normal range. Upon being notified, Dr. B. ordered a bronchodilator and, after assessing Esther a few minutes later, ordered that 500 cc of IV fluid be given all at once. There was no change in her blood pressure. At 12:30 p.m., approximately two hours after admission to the PACU, Dr. Y. ordered another 250 cc of IV fluid be given over 10 minutes. The nurses' progress notes document both orders for fluid, but do not indicate if they were given.

An electrocardiogram (ECG) done some time before 11:40 a.m. revealed an abnormality that could have been a result of cardiac problems, drugs or a decreased potassium level.

Approximately four hours after admission to the PACU, blood work showed that Esther had a low potassium level. She was then given potassium with her IV fluids. A few minutes later, a persistent cough, a symptom consistent with fluid in the lungs, was noted. Her oxygen saturation had dropped to 87 percent (low). She was administered oxygen and received bronchodilators and anti-nausea medication. Her total fluid balance, including what she had received in the operating room and the PACU, was a potential positive fluid balance of 3000 cc at 2:40 p.m.

At 3 p.m., Esther was returned to the ward. Her oxygen saturation level remained low. There is no indication in the documentation that a physician was made aware of her continuing low oxygen level. At 5:15 p.m., Esther's pulse rate rose to 120 beats per minute and it was irregular, a finding consistent with atrial fibrillation. Her chest was congested and her potassium and her oxygen saturation levels remained low.

A second ECG revealed atrial fibrillation and a high pulse rate of 155 beats per minute. Esther was attended by a resident physician and internist who prescribed medication to control her heart rate. Her oxygen saturation remained low at 88 percent. In the early evening, she was transferred to the intensive care unit.

At 10:30 p.m., Esther said she felt weak and had trouble breathing, but did not report experiencing chest pain. Her blood pressure fell and 40 minutes later it reached a critically low level of 73/40. She was given 500 cc of normal saline intravenously, which was followed by digoxin to control the atrial fibrillation. Blood tests for enzymes associated with myocardial infarction, a heart attack, showed a slight elevation. This elevation was not high enough to be diagnostic. Esther's oxygen saturation remained low in spite of being administered 100 percent oxygen.

Shortly after midnight on February 22, Esther became confused and within two hours was restless and appeared to have diminished mental capacity. At 3:24 a.m., a tube was placed in Esther's trachea, a process called intubation, and she was attached to a ventilator. Subsequently, her oxygen saturation level improved. At 3:27 a.m., Esther was cardioverted, a procedure by which an abnormally fast heart rate or cardiac arrhythmia is converted to normal using electricity or drugs. There was no documentation explaining why this was done.

Esther's severe hypotension (low blood pressure) continued through the early hours of February 22 in spite of treatment. Close to 4:30 a.m., she was given Lasix to promote urine output, but no written indication of why this was done exists. The internist called Lawrence at 4:30 a.m. to say things were serious and the family should come. Upon arrival at the hospital, Catherine, her father and brother, Ron, were told Esther was in critical condition and that she could have had a "silent" heart attack.

Throughout the remainder of February 22, Esther's condition remained relatively stable with the administration of medications to normalize her blood pressure, pulse and heart rate. On February 23, she continued to receive various medications and was started on a bowel care protocol. At this stage, Esther's physicians continued to suspect she had suffered a myocardial infarction.

On February 24, Esther was removed from the ventilator, the medications used to control the contractions of her heart muscles were administered orally rather than through an IV line, and an epidural drip for better pain control was restarted. The next day, it was documented that Esther was confused, agitated and had a "facial droop," an indication of nerve damage, commonly seen with brain injury. Esther's condition improved somewhat. She did, however, have periods of agitation, confusion and abdominal discomfort.

On February 28, Esther was transferred from the ICU to a nursing unit and on March 1 to the activation ward. Esther's condition showed only slow progress. Reports to family of Esther's condition from visitors during this period varied from her sometimes being completely engaged in conversations to being confused at other times. One visitor spoke of Esther's concern about herself, saying that Esther had said she was not "all there."

The bowel protocol, which consisted of oral stool softeners and laxatives, was continued, but there was no record of a bowel movement.

On the morning of March 3, Esther fell and was found lying beside her bed. Initially, she complained of back pain. In the early hours of March 4, Esther received the sedative Ativan, via an order obtained by the nursing staff over the telephone from the on-call physician. A few hours later at 5:30 a.m., Esther was found lying on her side on the floor beside her bed. She did not respond when spoken to, her body was stiff, she had jerky hand movements and her pupils were dilated and non-reactive. Her condition improved over the next several minutes, but even in her improved state she seemed "vague" and her speech was slurred. There was still no mention in the records of Esther having a bowel movement. Esther was examined by a physician who ordered blood work and an abdominal x-ray.

Around noon on March 4, Esther's family arrived at the hospital. At first, Catherine did not recognize the near-naked woman strapped into a wheelchair with facial bruises and scabs, and a bleeding nose as her mother. Esther was desperately trying to get the strap off her abdomen and kept saying how much it hurt. A clear yellow fluid was coming from her nose. Esther was extremely agitated.

Catherine asked to speak with her mother's general practitioner. She was told he was away for the weekend and was being replaced by another physician, Dr. R., who had not previously met Esther. He said he had examined her after the fall earlier that day and she had checked out okay. In response to Catherine's concerns about her mother's unusual and disconcerting behaviour, the physician said it was due to a combination of the surgery, multiple medications and anesthetic.

Catherine then enquired of the nurses about the medications her mother was receiving. She was surprised to learn that Tylenol 3 was among them. Esther had a history of Tylenol 3 interfering with normal bowel functioning.

In the afternoon of March 4, Esther told Catherine how much her stomach hurt and cried to get out of the wheelchair. Catherine cradled and rocked her mother. "Her stomach was now three times normal for her size. She kept complaining of being very sore there. Still there was no nursing staff or assistance," Catherine wrote in her journal.

In the late afternoon, Dr. R. assessed Esther, noting that she continued to be confused and to have abdominal pain. He told Catherine he was very concerned. Catherine wrote, "He told me then that there had been Ativan that he had not known about, and that this might have caused some of the behaviour of the night before. He ordered blood tests stat, an x-ray and instructed the nursing staff clean her up and put her to bed."

At 11 p.m. that night, Dr. R. called Catherine at home to say that they had an abdominal catastrophe on their hands. He had consulted with the on-call surgeon and together they had decided not to do emergency surgery in view of Esther's history and current instability. She would be given fluids and antibiotics intravenously. A CT scan was scheduled for the morning. Esther died four hours later at 3 a.m., March 5, 2000.

Questions, Wall of Silence and Turning Point

On Monday, March 6, Esther's family met with the general practitioner who said he was shocked to learn of Esther's death. When he had examined Esther on the previous Friday, he thought she was improving. He attributed the memory lapses to Esther's postoperative state, a common occurrence, in his opinion. The general practitioner agreed with the family's request for an autopsy to help find answers to their many questions. From the beginning, Catherine, her father and her brother did not want to lay blame. Rather, they wanted to find out why there had been an apparent lack of concern about Esther's care and what went wrong with the care itself. They also felt they had received mixed messages.

Catherine contacted the Coroners Service of British Columbia and learned that there are two types of autopsies. The purpose of a coroner's autopsy is to determine the cause of death. A hospital autopsy is performed on individuals for whom the cause of death is already known. The purpose of a hospital autopsy is to determine the extent of the disease and/or the effect of therapy and the presence of any undiagnosed condition that might have contributed to death.

The coroner's service authorized an autopsy as an initial step in its investigation. The autopsy determined the immediate cause of Esther's death to be ischemia (inadequate blood supply to an area resulting in shortage of oxygen) and infarction (death of tissue caused by lack of oxygen) of the bowel and brain. The cause of the ischemia and resulting infarction was the prolonged period of low blood pressure and low oxygen saturation levels following surgery. Esther also had fractured ribs and a closed head injury, known as a subdural hematoma, as a result of a fall. Evidence for a myocardial infarction was not found.

Catherine and her family continued their search for answers. She deluged officials with letters, writing to the health region board chair and members, surgeons, anesthetists, hospital administrators and heads of professional groups. For a long time Catherine did not receive one reply or even an acknowledgement. The wall of silence was deafening.

The Wincklers began to think that the legal, adversarial route was the only way to get answers to their questions. Lawyers had told them that they could look forward to years in court with a final settlement of only a few thousand dollars, perhaps $5,000, because that was the financial worth of a 77-year-old woman in British Columbia at the time. And that was only if they actually won, the likelihood of which was slim indeed. The doctors and hospital would be backed by the Canadian Medical Protective Association with resources of literally billions of dollars and a record of winning almost all of its cases.

As the family wavered in their deliberation about legal action, three events occurred, all near or shortly after the second anniversary of Esther's death, that convinced them to persist in working with the health-care system.

The first event came about as a result of Catherine having established the website EsthersVoice.com a year after her mother's death. Initially, this website was a way of telling Esther's family and many friends across Canada about what had happened to her, but in time it also became a place to share resources for families going through similar experiences. The goal from the beginning was to help ensure that what had happened to Esther would not happen to others.

The Wincklers were encouraged when a man wrote to them saying that because he had visited the website he had insisted that doctors attend to his mother whose symptoms they attributed to "senility." He strongly suspected that some medical condition was responsible for his mother's sudden onset of symptoms. Investigations revealed a 70 percent blockage of an important artery which likely would have caused the woman's death in weeks. The woman recovered and returned to active life.

Two subsequent events, the release of the results of the coroner's investigation and a series of prominent articles in the *Vancouver Sun* newspaper, affirmed the Wincklers' decision to continue a co-operative approach.

Coroner's Report and *Vancouver Sun*

Released more than two years after Esther's death, the report prepared by Coroner Margaret Turner ruled death as "accidental," which is defined by the coroner's service as a death caused by unnatural injuries. The purpose of a coroner's investigation is to find facts, not fault. In her report dated May 6, 2002, the coroner reported significant issues in 10 areas leading up to Esther's death. The report is available at EsthersVoice.com.

On the website, Catherine summarized these findings as broken ribs, concussion, malnutrition, dehydration, blocked bowels and improper documentation. She emphasized that no one had noticed that Esther had not had a bowel movement in 15 days.

The coroner's 10 areas of concern are stated and summarized below.

1. No documentation on the available health records related to the types of anesthesia discussed or consented to during the preoperative assessments.

Dr. B., the anesthetist who conducted the preoperative assessment the evening before surgery, told the coroner that he was aware of the first preoperative assessment in which it was concluded that a spinal anesthetic be used. Based on his expertise, however, Dr. B. decided to use a general rather than a spinal anesthetic. The reasons for this decision are not documented. Dr. B. claimed that Esther was very anxious about being awake during the surgery and that it was her wish to be put to sleep during the procedure. No documentation of this conversation exists. This claim was in stark contrast to the message Esther left on Catherine's answering machine following Dr. B.'s assessment. The Guidelines to the Practice of Anaesthesia recommended by the Canadian Anaesthetists' Society states that the details of the preoperative assessment should be documented on the patient's chart.

The coroner raised a related issue of signed consent, which means that the patient is aware of the procedure to be performed and its inherent risks. A consent for surgery was signed by Esther, the surgeon and a witness. The consent form, however, had no place to indicate what type of anesthesia the patient was consenting to. As well, the form was not dated, making it impossible to know when Esther gave consent and to what type of anesthetic.

2. Postoperative congestive heart failure was not identified and/or not treated promptly, although Esther exhibited signs and symptoms consistent with this condition.

Congestive heart failure (CHF) occurs when the heart is unable to adequately circulate the blood, resulting in fluid buildup in the lungs, which in turn depresses the patient's oxygen saturation. Esther showed symptoms consistent with CHF, in particular restlessness, feelings of unease, increased heart rate, low blood pressure and low oxygen saturation, fluid in the lungs and atrial fibrillation. The coroner did not find any documentation that most of these early signs were reported to the physician.

Esther received treatment that included administration of fluid, medication for atrial fibrillation and treatment to increase her blood pressure. However, treatment to decrease the fluid in her lungs did not begin until her oxygen saturation level had been at a critical level for more than 12 hours. The coroner wrote: "If the presence of congestive heart failure had been identified in the PACU (at the onset of the signs and symptoms suggesting an oxygen delivery problem) and treatment had been aimed directly at decreasing the pulmonary edema, then it is possible that Ms. Winckler may not have experienced the deterioration and complications that led to her death."

3. Medical management of a patient experiencing critically low oxygen levels and prolonged hypotension.
Investigations revealed that the autopsy findings of areas of ischemia and infarction in the colon and brain were a result of prolonged oxygen desaturation and hypotension in the postoperative period. In the immediate postoperative period, Esther had a low oxygen saturation for longer than 12 hours and low blood pressure for approximately seven hours. She was then placed on relatively high doses of epinephrine and dopamine for approximately two days. These medications, if used for prolonged periods or inappropriately, can lead to ischemia and possibly infarction of tissues.

Esther's signs and symptoms of a cerebral event on February 25 and 26 may have been a result of ischemia and/or infarction in the brain. As well, abdominal distension, pain and lack of bowel movements, which could have been caused by constipation, could also have been caused by ischemia and/or infarction of the bowel.

4. Documentation on the health records at the general hospital.
Although communication processes were in place at the general hospital to ensure appropriate flow of information, there were many instances during Esther's hospitalization where written documentation was lacking, inaccurate and/or incomplete. Both nursing and medical staff were involved in the poor documentation. As the coroner indicated, these may seem like minor errors, but they are significant

because poor communication can potentially lead to errors. (Poor communication can be considered an error in itself.)

Of particular relevance to Esther's case were the sporadic entries on the bowel movements section of the bowel care record and charting in regard to fluid administration. A result of the latter was that the fluid balance, a vital part of postoperative assessment, was incorrect by at least 750 cc. Fluid overload as observed in fluid in the lungs is a sign of congestive heart failure.

5. *Transfer of an unstable postoperative patient to an understaffed activation ward.*
On March 1, Esther was transferred from the surgical ward to an activation ward. In general, a patient on an activation ward has recovered from the acute stage of their health concern and is close to being discharged. Each nurse on an activation ward is responsible for a greater number of patients than on an acute care ward. Hospital staff told the coroner that Esther was transferred to the activation ward so soon after her postoperative difficulties because of a shortage of nurses on the surgical ward. The coroner raised the possibility that had Esther remained on the surgical ward her deterioration may have been identified earlier. She may have benefited from the surgical nurses' experience with common postoperative problems and the lower nurse-to-patient ratio on the surgical ward.

6. *No protocol for assessment of patients receiving analgesics and sedation.*
Protocols for managing patients receiving pain medication are commonly used in British Columbia hospitals. These protocols include documentation of respiratory rate, heart rate and blood pressure. Sedation and the effects of analgesics are recorded using standardized scales. The coroner was unable to find documentation that any protocol was used to assist in managing Esther's discomfort. Inappropriately managed pain can have a detrimental effect on the patient's physical condition, behaviour, mental state and recovery time. The coroner mentioned that poor pain management may have

contributed to some of Esther's restlessness and confusion that led to her two falls.

7. Providing for the nutritional needs of a patient recovering from surgery.
The coroner states that it appears Esther did not receive any nutrition before her condition became critical on February 22, the day after surgery. She is recorded to have had sips of fluid on February 24, eaten poorly on February 25, and eaten with assistance the next day. There is no documentation after the morning of February 28, when another diet order was written, that indicates Esther was receiving adequate nutrition. The coroner wrote that if Esther's diet was not adequate for her needs, this lack could have contributed to her "overall health status by decreasing her strength, impairing her immune system, impairing her respiratory drive, impairing her mental functioning and delaying the healing process."

8. Recognition, documenting and reporting of bowel movements, or lack of bowel movements.
Constipation is a common occurrence that has many causes ranging from something as simple as inadequate diet to a potentially fatal situation such as a bowel obstruction. From February 28 to March 5, there was no documentation related to diet, so it was impossible for the coroner to determine if Esther was eating a diet adequate to promote bowel function.

Esther was placed on a bowel protocol for six days beginning on February 27. None of the medications that were ordered during this time were documented as having been administered, despite the fact that Esther did not have a bowel movement for the entire six days the protocol was in place. Only seven of more than 36 boxes to be completed in the section to record bowel movements were completed. The coroner reported that if the staff had been following the bowel protocol appropriately, they may have identified Esther's abdominal problems sooner.

9. Recognition, and reporting, of abnormal signs indicative of a head injury.

Esther underwent physical and neuro-vital sign assessments after her fall on March 4. She exhibited a number of abnormal signs consistent with a serious head injury, including dilated and non-reactive pupils. She was unresponsive to verbal stimuli and displayed a stiff body, jerky hand movements, slurred speech and vagueness. There was bruising to the right side of her head. The autopsy revealed a recently sustained closed head injury in the same area of her head that had been injured in the fall. Esther's condition improved within 15 minutes of the fall, but her speech remained slurred. Further diagnostics which would have led to prompt treatment of a potentially fatal injury were not conducted.

10. Overall management of an elderly patient in the general hospital.
The coroner pointed out that several areas of care provided to Esther illustrated gaps between the standards that were recommended in the field of geriatrics at the time and those in use at the general hospital. These areas included pain management, effects of surgery on the geriatric patient, restraints, sedation, and nutrition and elimination. Esther would have had the best opportunity for recovery if practices in these areas had been conducted at a higher level, according to the coroner, who also wrote that some of the patient-care practices may have actually exacerbated Esther's condition.

The coroner made recommendations arising from the 10 areas of concern. These recommendations were sent to the Department of Anaesthesia and PACU, Patient Care Services and Acute and Strategic Services of the general hospital and to the Fraser Valley Health Region. She also recommended to the Registered Nurses' Association of BC that it consider offering an educational workshop at the hospital involving nursing care issues. A copy of the coroner's report was sent to the College of Physicians and Surgeons of BC to review for educational purposes as deemed appropriate.

On May 22, 2002, the day after Catherine gave the coroner's report to the *Vancouver Sun*, the newspaper ran a front page article, "Woman's Illness Injuries Went Untreated; Coroner: She Died after

Routine Hip Surgery." In the article, the Winckler family said that Esther's experience is a bellwether case that illustrates the plight of seniors in the health-care system.

Two additional articles appeared in the first section of the same issue. The first, "Daughter's Diary of Mom's Death," began, "During the final 15 days of Esther Winckler's life, her daughter, Catherine Winckler, kept a journal about her mother's treatment at Chilliwack Hospital. These are excerpts from that hospital journal, which the daughter submitted to the investigating coroner." It gives a heart-wrenching account as recorded by Catherine of her mother's hospitalization. On February 21, 2000, Catherine wrote that Esther had told her that the general practitioner "had assured her that *everyone* at the hospital knows about your case and not to worry, they were not going to take any chance and would do the spinal."

In the second article, "Daughter Hopes Her Mother's Story Will Be Heard," Catherine explained why she named the website Esther's Voice. "The coroner said they [coroners] were there, not to act for doctors, the nurses, the hospital, the police, or even the family. They were there to be Esther's voice — to hear the story that she had to tell us in death, the story she was incapable of telling us over her 15-day stay at Chilliwack General."

Several letters to the editor in response to Esther's story were published. Among them was a letter published on May 24 from a West Vancouver woman who congratulated Catherine on keeping such detailed notes and having the skills to effectively present the information. She also wrote that by sharing her mother's story, Catherine may have helped save lives.

Responding to Esther's Voice

The publicity coupled with the Winckler family's rejection of legal action set in motion responses that continue to save lives in British Columbia, across Canada and elsewhere. The Registered Nurses Association of BC (RNABC) was the first to contact Catherine. The RNABC asked two clinical nurse specialists (CNS), Pamela Ottem and Phyllis Hunt, to investigate. (The RNABC is now known as the College of Registered Nurses of BC.) They were joined by Marcia Carr, whom Cathy Weir, Quality Improvement and Patient Safety Officer for Fraser Health, had asked to work with Hunt at the general hospital. On May 23, the day after the story broke, an article in the *Vancouver Sun* announced that Chilliwack General Hospital was set-ting up a multi-disciplinary committee to review the coroner's report and would meet with the family.

Hunt and Carr found nurses at the hospital eager to learn how to avoid the types of errors that played a role in Esther's death. Once they recognized the extent of the nurses' lack of knowledge, Hunt and Carr sought the assistance of two other clinical nurse special-ists, one from Providence Health Care and the other from Vancouver Coastal Health. During the following year, they expanded their group, obtained funding from the Ministry of Health Nursing Directorate for travel and materials, and developed workshops. Their next achieve-ment was launching the Acute Care Geriatric Nurse Network (ACGNN).

Founded in 2003, the ACGNN is a collaboration between the province's Nursing Directorate, clinical nurse specialists with exper-tise in various aspects of elder care, and geriatrics and home health professionals for the five health authorities. The network is dedicated to improving care for acutely ill older adults, wherever they may be in the continuum of care.

By April 2004, ACGNN included 11 clinical nurse specialists, senior care experts who work in all health authority regions of the province. In 2001, there had been only three such specialists. By June 2004, the organization had trained 627 nurses. Carr estimated that four years later approximately 1,500 nurses in BC had upgraded the skills they need to care for elderly patients. "However, I hon-estly cannot say how many across Canada, the United States and the United Kingdom have been made aware of Esther and the ACGNN, because of the websites," Carr said. At the end of the workshops, which were presented throughout the province, participants were encouraged to contact the clinical specialists for help in future cases.

This connection has proven to be especially important for nurses in remote communities.

Helping people navigate the health-care system is a major goal in the work undertaken by Carr and her colleagues. "It's a black hole for many, even for those working in the system," she said. ACGNN helps nurses, elders and their families make their way through the system. "If you don't know what you don't know, how do you know what to ask?" Carr said. In response to the many emails and calls she receives from concerned families, Carr does not give advice; rather, she suggests key questions people can ask care providers.

Over the next three years, members of ACGNN realized that most older adults enter the health-care system through emergency rooms. Accurate assessment by triage nurses is crucial to patients receiving appropriate care. "It's critical for acute care staff to be able to recognize the atypical ways older patients present. Symptoms, vitals and lab work can be different than for young patients," Carr said. She added that 92 percent of the older population live in the community rather than a care facility. "Acute care should only be an episodic glitch. If treated correctly, the patients should be out of hospital quickly and back home," Carr said.

Soon Carr and colleagues established the Geriatric Emergency Nursing Initiative (GENI). With additional funding from the Nursing Directorate, two-day workshops were developed. A GENI e-learning module was also developed and a binder of prompt cards produced. The cards focus on what is known as the "Geriatric Giants," including delirium, dementia, depression, incontinence, falls, constipation, pain and unsettled behaviour.

The ACGNN workshops were held for six years and the GENI program for three. In March 2008, funding for travel ended, which forced Carr and colleagues to turn to distance learning tools to deliver the workshop material. Many resources are available on the website, acgnn.ca, including the GENI lectures. The website is operated by the clinical nursing specialists on their own time. During the operation of the in-person workshops, the CNSs, all with full-time jobs, used many hours of personal time to make the ACGNN program happen. "It's absolutely essential to keep improving what we do and to keep people safe and cared for," Carr said.

Carr, Hunt and colleagues continue to use Esther's death as a teaching tool. Telling the story of a real person is an excellent way to get people's attention and to illustrate the types of problems that can occur, especially with older patients. A link to *Esther's Story: Health System in Failure, Hope for the Future* appears on the home page of the network's website. Representatives of Fraser Health and the ACGNN CNSs tell Esther's story wherever possible, including in staff orientations and at regional and national conferences.

As part of an interdisciplinary team from the University of British Columbia faculties of medicine, nursing and allied health professions, Carr has played an instrumental role in the development of modules within the university's Care for Elders Program. The role of the program, which was funded originally in 2002 from the BC Ministry of Health through its Strategic Teaching Initiative, is to integrate findings from studies about care for elders into service delivery. Education reaches students across the spectrum, from undergraduate to postgraduate to continuing education. The program has developed 16 interdisciplinary case-based educational modules that can be used anywhere in British Columbia. Carr is an active participant in many of the modules, which deal with topics such as communication and hearing loss in elders, incontinence and falls.

Carr was particularly encouraged by a recent intergenerational conference. Students of medicine and nursing and those in allied fields, such as occupational health, had the opportunity to hear seniors' points of view. Carr stressed the importance of the participation of these healthy and active seniors. "Health-care providers usually see older people in acute-care situations," she said.

Reflecting on the decade since the release of the coroner's report and coverage by the *Vancouver Sun*, Carr said, "Esther's story and the family's approach give us hope that by working together in a constructive way, we as health-care providers can improve care and support for older adults. The Wincklers' insistence not to let this happen to anyone else gave us the pivotal story we needed to move forward."

Fraser Health implemented policies to use fewer restraints and to inform patients or families when mistakes have been made. Fraser Health's Geriatric Clinical Services Planning and Delivery team partnered with ACGNN to produce additional e-learning modules. In 2008, Abbotsford Regional Hospital, the first hospital built in the province specifically designed to be elder-friendly, opened its doors. At least five BC hospitals have units for acute care of the elderly.

In contrast to Fraser Health and the RNABC, the College of Physicians and Surgeons of BC did not see opportunities for improvement. The case, as presented in the coroner's report, never went past peer review for any follow-up practice recommendations or to the disciplinary committee. This was a great disappointment to the Winckler family, who had hoped that removing the possibility of litigation would open avenues for honest dialogue, disclosure and recognition of responsibility that would assist physicians in providing better care.

Many thousands of people from around the world continue to hear Esther's voice. Catherine receives calls and emails from nurses and families from across Canada and overseas. The director of a long-term care institution in Montreal wrote to say that Esther's story is discussed as a learning experience for nurses working in the facility. The website is required reading in many courses for nurses. Recently, a registered nurse in Ontario who was enrolled in a critical care course sent Catherine an email which included these thoughts: "After reading your Mom's story, I can honestly say that I will be a better nurse and will advocate even more than I already do. I find myself with the attitude that I treat all my patients with the same care I would expect for myself or my own family. I admire your efforts to direct your energy toward change. Your website will save and change lives. I didn't know your Mom, but I am certain she would be very proud."

Catherine's response to the nurse concluded with these words: "I often get emails from a family who is either facing the impending death of a loved one, or has lost someone, and finds our site and wonders what to do. I can't give them advice; I can only share our story. Each person's journey is very different and for some, a lawsuit is the only way they will find satisfaction. In our case, every time I receive a letter like yours I know that we did the right thing by just sharing every single thing, and not settling anything behind closed doors. My mum would be proud; I am starting to see that more and more. So, on behalf of the surviving Winckler family — thank you."

The Winckler family is establishing a trust in Esther's name to provide financial assistance to nursing students interested in the area of geriatrics. By helping students, the trust will honour Esther's love of education.

Commenting on what her family has learned, Catherine says that patience is essential, as is the need to separate grief from pursuing justice. She also says it is essential to learn about the systems involved in order to be able to navigate them successfully. Catherine emphasizes the importance of not relying on others to accomplish what you can do. Take the lead! She did and with results beyond anything she could have ever imagined.

Heartbeat

For several years after the sudden death of her teenaged son in 1990 from a misdiagnosed inherited cardiac arrhythmia, Pam Husband was told by members of the medical community that such deaths were rare. But upon hearing frequent mention of sudden, unexplained deaths of young people in casual social conversations, her instinct and intellect told her otherwise. Today, inherited cardiac arrhythmias are recognized as one of the leading causes of death of Canadians under 35 years of age. Over the same period, the number of these types of disorders known to medical science has more than tripled.

In 1995, Pam and Dr. Robert Hamilton of Toronto's Hospital for Sick Children decided to form a group which has evolved into the Canadian Sudden Arrhythmia Deaths Syndrome (SADS) Foundation. Pam and the foundation play major roles in the support of patients and families, providing educational opportunities and raising awareness. They also advocate for research to improve diagnosis and treatments of these diseases, often working closely with medical researchers and policy makers.

In 1990, Pam Husband's 16-year-old son, Greg, was found dead in his bed. He was discovered by his father who had gone to awaken him. But Greg didn't wake up. Greg's sudden, unexpected death was all the more devastating for his family because the cause could not be identified.

As a child, Greg had fainting spells when he was startled. He would pass out at the sound of the alarm clock and once fainted when he got off a ride at an amusement park. Doctors told Greg's parents that his electrocardiogram (ECG) result was normal and their son had epilepsy of unknown causes.

Greg's younger sister, Leigh, also passed out occasionally, but the triggers for her loss of consciousness were more diverse than her brother's had been. Simply being very tired could result in Leigh fainting. After Greg's death, Leigh had several fainting spells, which prompted Pam to seek further medical help. The general practitioner referred them to a neurologist who thought the problem could be associated with Leigh's heart. He sent them to see a cardiologist.

Eighteen months after Greg's death, Leigh was diagnosed as having Long QT syndrome. This condition is caused by episodes of abnormalities in the heart's electrical system associated with an irregular heartbeat originating from the ventricles. These episodes may lead to palpitations, fainting and sudden death because of ventricular fibrillation. Various types of stimuli may initiate episodes. The condition is called Long QT because the QT interval on electrocardiograms is longer than normal.

Pam retrieved Greg's ECG that had been done two years before his death. Upon examination, an expert electrophysiologist-cardiologist said that the ECG indicated Greg had a prolonged QT interval, and most likely suffered from LQTS. This condition, being electrical in nature, was not detected at autopsy because the heart tissue looked normal. The coroner's investigation did not include a re-examination of the ECG in Greg's medical records. "In hindsight, my son's symptoms seemed pretty obvious," Pam said.

When Leigh was first diagnosed, members of the Canadian medical community repeatedly told Pam that LQTS was extremely rare. The cardiologist who diagnosed Leigh said that hers was the first case of Long QT syndrome he had seen in his 40 years of practice. Pam recalled asking him, "How many have you missed?" From this point forward, Pam suspected that cases of LQTS occured much more frequently than had been recognized by the medical community. At social events, she kept hearing about other families whose young sons and daughters had died suddenly from unexplained causes.

In 1994, Pam learned of an American organization called Sudden Arrhythmia Death Syndromes (SADS) Foundation through a LQTS registry in Rochester, New York. "That summer the American SADS group sent me newspaper articles about families who had experienced similar sudden deaths," Pam said. She then contacted the *Toronto Star* newspaper, which ran a feature article about Greg and LQTS over the 1994 Thanksgiving weekend.

Almost 300 families from across Canada telephoned in response to the article. Pam's suspicion about the prevalence of heart arrhythmias was confirmed. "I had no plan at the time I contacted the *Star*. I simply wanted to talk to another mother who had been through what I was going through," Pam said. She has subsequently learned that several Canadians were diagnosed with LQTS as a result of the article.

Pam experienced distinct differences in the responses by some cardiologists who treated adults and by cardiologists who cared for children. Members of the former group accused Pam of inciting panic in the Canadian population and assured her that inherited cardiac arrhythmic disorders could never affect a significant percentage of the population. In contrast, pediatric cardiologists were generally receptive to considering the importance of arrhythmias. Pam attributes this difference to pediatricians usually dealing with a third party, parents, and thinking of medical conditions in a more holistic family-centred way.

In January 1995, more than 100 people attended a meeting which Pam had organized at a Mississauga hotel. The group, including Dr. Robert Hamilton of the Hospital for Sick Children and Pam, decided to create a national charitable organization. At first, they thought it would be a small parental support group. However, it quickly evolved into the Canadian Sudden Arrhythmia Death Syndromes Foundation. Initially, the Canadian group relied on its American counterpart, but soon became a strong vibrant organization in its own right. Within two years, the Canadian SADS Foundation had a mailing list of more than 1,200. Dr. Hamilton continues to serve on the SADS medical advisory board.

The American SADS Foundation had its beginning in the early 1970s when Dr. Michael Vincent and his colleagues at the LDS Hospital and the University of Utah in Salt Lake City were studying LQTS. They were particularly interested in familial histories. Many LQTS patients were identified and one particularly large family became the world's largest single LQTS pedigree.

In 1988, geneticist Dr. Ray White and his colleagues at the University of Utah partnered with Dr. Vincent in order to find the genetic abnormality in this largest of LQTS families. A year later, Dr. Mark Keating joined the faculty at the university and began the genetic studies that lead in 1991 to the report of the genetic location for the LQTS gene on chromosome 11. This discovery was met with considerable excitement and interest in both the medical community and the general public.

Despite significant advances in research and reports in the medical literature, it appeared to Dr. Vincent that too few physicians were familiar with or tested for LQTS. He said "there must be a better way" to spread information about LQTS, and save the lives of children and young adults. In December 1991, the Sudden Arrhythmia Death Syndromes Foundation was established by Dr. Vincent, several colleagues and LQTS family members. The purpose of the organization was to save the lives and support the families of children and young adults who are genetically predisposed to sudden death due to heart rhythm abnormalities.

The Canadian SADS Foundation was established in 1995 and the U.K. SADS Foundation in 2000. Subsequently, SADS foundations or groups with similar goals have been started in other countries, including Australia and South Africa.

Today, Canadian SADS operates a wide spectrum of programs and projects under the direction of a board of directors with the assistance of a medical advisory board. The foundation's headquarters is an office in Pam's home. Everyone is a volunteer, including Pam, president and executive director, who averages 30 hours a week on SADS-related work. Funding for the foundation comes from donations from individuals, corporations and other foundations.

From the beginning, Pam approached the development of the SADS Foundation as a business. "I understand the business model. Even though SADS is non-profit, the concept is the same as for a for-profit business," she said. A former teacher turned certified management consultant, Pam ran her own business to train people how to operate computer accounting systems for a number of years. Her ability to work with many types of people has also contributed significantly to the success of the Canadian SADS Foundation.

The foundation is committed to delivering three core services: support for patients and families affected by an inherited cardiac rhythm disorder, education and awareness of the warning signs for these disorders among primary-care physicians and all adults who care for and work with children, and encouragement of research to improve diagnosis and treatment of these disorders.

Establishment and maintenance of the foundation's website, sads. ca, ranks high on Pam's list of priorities. The website provides visitors with information about arrhythmia disorders, warning signs, and events and conferences. Links to related sites and information on supporters and fundraisers are also available. Brochures in French and English and periodic newsletters can be downloaded. There are also information booklets for patients and families affected by SADS. The website also provides a forum for families affected by SADS to share their stories.

Recently, Canadian SADS, with financial support from the Ontario Trillium Foundation, produced a YouTube video (youtube. com/user/TheCANSADS) that is generating considerable interest. The video emphasizes the importance of the three warning signs of cardiac arrhythmias.

- Fainting (syncope) or seizure during physical activity,
- Fainting or seizure associated with excitement, emotional stress or startle,
- Family history of unexpected sudden death during physical activity or during a seizure, or any other unexplained sudden death of an otherwise healthy young person.

Dr. Joel Kirsh, a pediatric cardiologist at Toronto's Hospital for Sick Children who also serves on the SADS medical advisory board, stresses in the video the importance of recognizing these signs and acting upon them. About half of the 700 to 900 Canadians under the age of 35 who die annually from inherited arrhythmias have displayed at least one warning sign.

In 2010, Ms. Emily Ballantyne and Dr. Andrew Krahn of the Arrhythmia Service, Division of Cardiology, University of Western Ontario, released a paper, *The Scope and Impact of Inherited Cardiac Rhythm Disorders in Canada*. The document was created at the request of the Canadian SADS Foundation to provide resource information regarding the scope and impact of inherited cardiac rhythm disorders in Canada. Dr. Krahn is a member of the SADS medical advisory board.

Ms. Ballantyne and Dr. Krahn reported that more Canadians under 35 die from sudden cardiac arrest than from all childhood cancers combined. One type of inherited cardiac abnormality, Wolff-Parkinson White syndrome, occurs at the same prevalence in Canadian children as cystic fibrosis. As many as one in 500 people are estimated to have a type of cardiac arrhythmia, known as hypertrophic cardiomyopathy. Dr. Kirsh said this means that in a large high school of 1,000 enrolment, two students could be at risk because of this one disorder alone.

Susan Csatari, a registered nurse and SADS board member, encourages parents who think their child may have any of the SADS symptoms to immediately seek medical attention for a cardiac assessment. Her son, Stephen, 20, a university student and athlete, collapsed and died in 2002 while running on a country road. Susan later learned that he had once passed out while jogging.

The specific cause of Stephen's death was arrhythmogenic right ventricular cardiomyopathy (AVRC), which is one of a growing number of recognized inherited cardiac arrhythmias that can cause sudden death. When Pam's son died, only three were known. The SADS website provides information on the various arrhythmias which fall into two general groups — those that interfere with the muscle system of the heart and those that cause malfunctioning of the heart's electrical system.

If diagnosed, inherited arrhythmias are treatable and manageable. Treatment varies with individuals and their conditions, and often involves medications. Positive results are verified by participants in the SADS YouTube video. Donata Leuenberger was diagnosed with CPVT (catecholaminergic polymorphic ventricular tachycardia) at age 10 and her son, Simon, at age 5. Simon takes medications several times a day and has regular checkups, including ECGs. Mother and son both live active, full lives. After being told in the emergency room that her pounding heart was nothing to worry about, Micayla Ahearn, a gifted figure skater, was diagnosed with LQTS. "You can lead more than a normal life. You can live a beautiful life," she said. Micayla is among the lucky ones whose original misdiagnosis did not prove fatal.

In contrast, Jessica Barnett died of an inherited arrhythmia following misdiagnosis. After a five-year history of fainting and being incorrectly diagnosed with idiopathic epilepsy, Jessica died at age 17 of LQTS. Her mother, Tanya, recalled on the YouTube video that several months before her death, Jessica was told by a physician that "you need to go home and learn to breathe through this." After her death, Jessica's father was diagnosed with LQTS and prescribed medication. He now has an implanted defibrillator.

With Jessica, Pam's son and many others, the error in diagnosis was discovered after death. The question arises, however, of how many sudden, unexplained deaths could have been from misdiagnosed or undiagnosed arrhythmias. Inherited arrhythmias may account for such incidents as sudden drowning and as the cause of some otherwise unexplained motor vehicle accidents. Research supports that SADS may be involved in some SIDS (sudden infant death syndrome) cases.

All of the members of the Canadian SADS board are affected in some way by SADS. Graham Davies, treasurer, was a close friend of Stephen Csatari. Nancy Busse, like Susan Csatari, lost a child to a cardiac arrhythmia. In 1999, Nancy's daughter, Susan Read, 23, herself the mother of a one-year-old boy, died in her sleep while on a family vacation. There was no apparent cause of death. Just two weeks before her death, Susan had passed a physical exam with flying colours.

After much investigation, Nancy came to the conclusion that

her daughter died from LQTS. The tip-off for Nancy came when she saw a TV drama about a young woman who died unexpectedly from LQTS. Nancy has continued to be a loyal supporter and to volunteer for the Canadian SADS Foundation since 1999.

In 2009, at the age of 27, Allison Larouche (née Cleland), board member and education coordinator, was diagnosed with ARVC. The former university basketball star collapsed while on a training run for her fourth marathon. She had shrugged off the periods of dizziness she had experienced on previous runs. Her running companion, a friend who had just finished medical school, insisted that Allison go to the ER. Within three months, she was diagnosed with ARVC. Allison's heart muscle was damaged to the point of interfering with the electrical system, so she had a defibrillator implanted as well as being prescribed beta blocker medications.

Allison is grateful for the quick diagnosis of the AVRC, which prevented her from participating in the marathon that might have proved fatal. She appreciates the ongoing care provided by Dr. Andrew Krahn, who closely monitors her condition and keeps her informed about advances related to inherited arrhythmias via frequent emails. "I'm lucky. Through my work with SADS, I've become aware of people who have had delayed or incorrect diagnoses," Allison said.

Having hung up her running shoes for good, Allison keeps in shape with yoga and cycling. Her husband, an orthopedic surgeon, helps her keep a careful watch on her level of exertion.

A physical education teacher in Toronto, Allison, who is also a consultant for the Ontario Physical Health Education Association (OPHEA), works toward increasing the awareness of SADS in schools and sporting organizations. Recently, thanks in large part to Allison, OPHEA instituted the policy that instructs teachers and others working with children to call 911 whenever a student faints, even for the first time.

SADS board director Robert Boudreau has experience with inherited cardiac rhythm abnormalities both in his personal life and in his work as a paramedic in Nova Scotia. "When we were getting ready to go on vacation, my son started feeling unwell. My wife, a registered nurse, found he had a very irregular heartbeat, so we took him to the ER," Robert said. A cardiologist diagnosed the boy with LQTS and recommended that other family members be tested as well. One of Robert's two daughters and his wife were subsequently found to have LQTS. In retrospect, Robert and his wife realized that she had been showing signs of LQTS for more than 20 years.

Robert joined the SADS board in 2011 after hearing a presentation given by Pam at a paramedics' conference. Robert now speaks to other paramedics and at various conferences across the country. Recently, he and Pam raised awareness of SADS at British Columbia's Justice Institute, which provides training for paramedics. Locally in Nova Scotia, Robert often speaks about SADS in schools and to paramedics in training.

Such education pays off. Pam recently received an email from a public access defibrillation coordinator in Western Canada telling of a paramedic who had attended a SADS information session. Not long after hearing about SADS, the paramedic was at a soccer game when he witnessed a young girl collapse while running on the field. She was not in cardiac arrest but had completely passed out. The parents thought the girl was okay, but the paramedic insisted that she be medically assessed. The coordinator wrote: "This is what we were aiming for in education. I was so excited I had to share it with someone. He [the paramedic] came by today and told me about it, and grabbed some more pamphlets to provide more information to the family to make sure they push to get the right answers."

In his own work as a paramedic, Robert responds to calls of faints and seizures resulting from a variety of causes. When a SADS warning sign is involved, such as fainting during physical activity, Robert and his colleagues consider this in the differential diagnosis. They treat and document any clinical signs and symptoms forming the clinical impression. These findings are included in the report to ER physicians. "We are saving lives," Robert said referring both to his work as a paramedic and his advocacy role for SADS.

Starting in 1999, the Canadian SADS Foundation has organized frequent conferences across the country. In 2011, the foundation hosted conferences called Living with Inherited Cardiac Rhythm Disorders in Ottawa and in Newtown, Newfoundland and Labrador. These conferences provide opportunities for individuals affected by inherited cardiac rhythm disorders and families who have experienced a sudden unexplained death of a young person to become proactive advocates for their own health. Health-care professionals, EMS personnel, teachers and amateur sports representatives benefit from the opportunity to learn of recent advances in research and to interact with other participants. Pam considers the conferences among the highlights of her work with the SADS Foundation. "It's wonderful to be with other people who 'get it,'" she said.

Other sources of satisfaction for Pam include the establishment of a database of 1,700 Canadian families. Another source is the interaction with the medical community, which she sees as a synergy benefiting both individuals affected by inherited arrhythmias and the medical community. Advances in research and treatment in the medical world provide encouragement for SADS volunteers. In return, the SADS Foundation can be a resource for patient research and advocacy.

In the years since Greg's death, Pam has seen major advances in research and treatment of SADS, as well as in the way sudden deaths are investigated. Molecular autopsy, a technique which examines the deceased's DNA, can determine if death was most likely caused by SADS. If such is the case, then family members can be tested, precautions taken and lives saved.

The Ontario coroner's service has proactively updated its guidelines for the investigation of sudden cardiac deaths of people between the ages two and 40. In the case of sudden premature deaths, investigating coroners must obtain all medical records, including cardiac investigations, especially ECGs, and establish a detailed family history of any sudden, unexplained or cardiac deaths. Pathologists who conduct autopsies on young sudden-death victims are required to store heart tissue for future genetic testing. Pam hopes to see the coroner services in other provinces adopt similar guidelines.

Research underway through Memorial University in St. John's

promises to provide answers for the sudden deaths through several centuries in many families and to save lives of members of the current and future generations. The research is focused on 16 extended kinships of close to 1,200 people, all of whom are thought to be linked to a common 18th-century ancestor. Family lore has arisen as a way of trying to explain these deaths of young people who died suddenly for no apparent reason, Pam said. These deaths were often recorded in family bibles, providing valuable information to researchers who think that ARVC was responsible. Many of the living family members have been diagnosed with ARVC and are receiving treatment. Contemplating parenthood, some of the younger members are considering in vitro fertilization and pre-implantation genetic embryo testing as a way to remove the ARVC gene from their family lineage and protect future generations.

Ms. Ballantyne and Dr. Krahn concluded their 2010 paper on the scope and impact of inherited cardiac rhythm disorders in Canada with an outline for continued success and these encouraging words.

> In order for patients to receive treatment in a timely fashion, health-care professionals must be educated and aware of these cardiac conditions. By continuing to train physicians in recognizing potential inherited cardiac rhythm disorder patients, the number of patients who are not diagnosed or misdiagnosed can be decreased. Conferences and seminars, as well as published articles discussing inherited cardiac rhythm disorders, are useful for providing information to health-care professionals.
>
> Likewise, increasing the general population's understanding of inherited cardiac rhythm disorders is a necessity for decreasing the number of sudden deaths in Canada. Media communication in newspapers, magazines, radio and television and the internet can help inform the public regarding inherited cardiac rhythm disorders. As individuals become aware of the signs and symptoms of these cardiac conditions, they are more likely to recognize and assist an individual who is suffering from an arrhythmic event.
>
> Additionally, public policy makers and health-care leaders play a

key role in directing attention and resources to detection and treatment of inherited cardiac rhythm disorders. An example is recent increased access to genetic testing to facilitate family screening and preventative therapy. This is a resource-intensive strategy that is strongly endorsed by physicians as a key preventative measure. These principles will be outlined in the forthcoming Canadian Cardiovascular Society/Canadian Heart Rhythm Society Recommendations for the Use of Genetic Testing in the Clinical Evaluation of Inherited Cardiac Arrhythmias Associated with Sudden Cardiac Death.

Public access to defibrillation technology and education regarding use of automatic external defibrillators (AEDs) will also enhance survival in cardiac arrest victims. By making AEDs accessible in public spaces, the chances of an individual receiving defibrillation in a timely fashion increases. In 2007–2008, the Government of Ontario installed 346 automated external defibrillators in government buildings. By continuing to provide AEDs in public locations, the number of cardiac arrest survivors will continue to rise.

For those with inherited cardiac rhythm disorders, the future looks promising. Genetic analysis allows for family members of affected individuals to be tested. If positive, treatment can be initiated before the onset of symptoms. Early diagnosis of inherited cardiac rhythm disorders and initiation of treatment may prevent fatal arrhythmic events. The continued funding and support of medical research, as well as the enhancement of public awareness of inherited arrhythmias ensures that the lives of those affected will continue to improve.

Thousands of Canadians with inherited cardiac arrhythmias whose lives have been saved and their families can thank Pam for understanding the power of the press and the power of the personal. She and her many dedicated associates have helped to make possible the statement "that the lives of those affected will continue to improve."

Take Action[1]

Beverley Williston's letter to the editor of a local newspaper is an example of how one person can take action to educate the public about medical errors.

To the Editor:

I would like to share with the public a couple of medical issues our family encountered in dealing with a loved one's illness.

If you or a loved one is sent for medical tests, scans, etc., please, please call and check on the results yourself, have them read in their entirety and do not wait to be called.

We are often told that if there's a problem we will be contacted, but that is not always the case, nor was it with our mother. A little over six months ago, we lost our mother to cancer. This disease in itself is horrible enough to deal with, but when errors are made along the way, it just adds insult to injury.

A small malignant tumour was inadvertently detected in our mother's lung during a routine abdominal/leg scan after a surgery and, although it was duly reported at the time, it somehow got overlooked and this cancer was not treated at its earliest stage.

After a similar scan some seven months later, this tumour was again reported and this time it was noted, but it had grown in size and had spread and we were told it was inoperable.

The bottom line here was that our mother was not given the opportunity for treatment at the earlier stage because of negligence.

We had assumed everything was fine because we had not received any call to the contrary, as our mother had several of these types of scans prior and all had been good, we had no reason to question it.

Obviously, our family was very upset by this mistake, but we did learn a disturbing fact from speaking with other families and even medical personnel. That fact was that these errors happen more than you can imagine. Doctors literally hold our lives in their hands, and although I realize they are human and can make mistakes, these types of errors are totally unacceptable, especially when these reports pass through many hands.

Someone should have picked up on this error.

Our mother did die from this cancer, and maybe this was her destiny and time, but I will never really know.

So, my message is to check on your test results and don't wait to be called.

You must be an advocate for yourself and your loved ones, and be very aware of what is medically happening around you.

If this letter can help only one family from experiencing the grief and anger that we felt because of such negligence, then it will be worth it.

The other issue we encountered speaks to those of you who may have a loved one living in independent seniors' housing where various services may be offered. Again, be an advocate to those people and ensure that the service, specifically if it involves dispensing of medicines, is being correctly administered to them, because mistakes can happen there as well.

Beverley Williston
Point-du-Chene

Over a year after writing the above letter, Beverley shared her reflections:

At the time I wrote my letter I was very angry and although many people tried to dissuade me from writing it, with comments such as "it won't make a difference anyway," "you won't beat them," etc., I felt that until I put words to my feelings and shared them with others I wouldn't be able to get past the anger. I felt I needed to do something, and since suing wasn't an option, I wanted people to know what had happened to us and maybe it could help someone else. Also, I hoped that maybe the doctor would read my letter and see himself, because he certainly knew who I was. Even today when I discuss what happened to my Mom to whomever will listen, I still get very agitated, and this probably won't ever go away.

In addition to writing to the paper, I tell anyone who will listen to make sure they check their test results and not wait for any doctor to call them. We waited with devastating results.

Some of the medical people I have spoken with say these types of errors are not uncommon, they happen a lot, but try to get them to admit the errors and they clam up.

The attending doctor to whom the radiologist's report was sent told my sister he was sorry our mother had cancer. However, he said it was not his fault the tumour had not been treated earlier, because, according to him, the detection of a small tumour had not been flagged in the radiologist's original report. The radiologist denied this accusation. I know for a fact that detection of the tumour was flagged, because I saw the report. Another doctor to whom a copy of the report had been sent told me he saw the flag and assumed the attending physician would take appropriate action.

The essential lessons to be learned from this story are that trusting your doctor is important, but blind faith can be deadly and you must be an advocate for yourself and your loved ones. If an error does occur, take action even if it's simply telling other people about your experience or writing a letter to a newspaper. Raising awareness through public education is a fundamental step toward the eventual goal of reducing the incidence of medical errors.

Not Too Late

Frank Gomberg

On October 21, 1998, 10-year-old Lisa Shore was admitted to the Hospital for Sick Children in Toronto because of severe pain in her leg. Her condition was not life-threatening, but rather a chronic disorder arising from a broken leg she had suffered eight months earlier. Upon Lisa's arrival at the emergency room, the attending physician administered morphine and then put her on a morphine pump. He entered his orders as to how Lisa should be monitored into a computer system in the emergency room. Nurses are supposed to check the system when a patient is taken to a room on a ward. The physician ordered that Lisa was to have her vital signs checked hourly and she was to be put on a Corometric monitor, a device that measures heart rate and respiration. The physician also ordered nurses to do a pain and sedation scale every hour in order to determine the level of Lisa's pain and drowsiness. The physician wrote on Lisa's chart that the nurses should check the computer for his orders.

Once Lisa was admitted to her room, the nurses neither checked the computer for orders nor referred to the protocol manual that tells nurses what to do if a child is on a morphine pump. They also did not do the hourly check of Lisa's vital signs or put Lisa on the Corometric monitor. Heavily drugged on morphine, Lisa fell asleep, as did Lisa's mother, Sharon, who was at her daughter's bedside. At 7 a.m. the next morning, October 22, 1998, Sharon was awakened when doctors making their rounds entered the room. They discovered Lisa was dead. An autopsy revealed that Lisa had most likely died of respiratory depression caused by the effects of morphine. The hospital did not contest the autopsy findings.

On September 30, 1999, a civil case between the Shore family and the hospital was settled before a mediator. On November 8, 1999, a coroner's inquest began which, upon its conclusion on February 24, 2000, resulted in 35 recommendations aimed at preventing similar deaths and the verdict that Lisa's death was a homicide. A Toronto police homicide squad launched an investigation. In 2001, Lisa's two nurses were charged with criminal negligence causing death, but the charges were withdrawn in 2003. In 2005, Lisa's nurses were found guilty of professional misconduct by their nursing licensing body. Immediately following this finding, the nurses returned to their jobs at the hospital.

Following Lisa's death, Sharon wrote a book, No Moral Conscience, about these events, describing how the hospital and its lawyers tried to cover up what had happened. She also established a website, LisaShore.com, with links to an exhaustive list of relevant documents, including newspaper articles and the inquest judgment. As a result of her experiences related to Lisa's death, Sharon entered Osgoode Hall Law School in September 2002 as a mature student. She was called to the Bar of Ontario in September 2006 and is now practicing law in Toronto.

Frank Gomberg, then a Toronto lawyer and now a full-time mediator, represented the Shore family from shortly after Lisa's death to completion of the inquest. As part of the requirements for his Master of Laws awarded by Osgoode Hall Law School in June 2011, Frank submitted a major research paper, "Apology for the Unexpected Death of a Child in a Healthcare Facility: A Prescription for Improvement." In this 129-page paper, Frank discusses the psychological dynamics arising from the wrongful death of a child and what constitutes an apology. He also discusses errors and adverse events within a health-care setting and apology, morality and law. Frank uses three case histories of the unexpected death of a child within a health-care facility as a teaching tool. Lisa Shore's case is among this trilogy. Frank's paper, including references substantiating his statements presented below, is available online.

The portion of Frank's paper concerning the Shore case is included here because timely, sincere apologies that acknowledge responsibility and express remorse help to reduce the adversarial aspects of the interaction between the family and the health-care facility. This in turn leads to an atmosphere not only of healing for families, but also one that is conducive to the study of the causes of errors and adverse events and their prevention.

Frank provides three quotations that summarize the importance of apology in health care.

> A stiff apology is a second insult . . . The injured party does not want to be compensated because he has been wronged; he wants to be healed because he has been hurt. — G.K. Chesterton

> The doctor who wants to get in trouble after an incident of actual malpractice can do so easily. All he has to do is avoid the patient, blame the patient for the bad result, refuse to talk to the family, refuse to apologize, refuse to listen in humility to patient castigation, and then to send his bill as usual. The doctor who wants to guarantee a breakdown in the relationship does not have to do all of the foregoing, just a few will suffice. The doctor who does not want to be sued will avoid these traps and will face the patient with humble sympathy and courage for the truth. — Ann J. Kellett, "Healing Angry Wounds," citing R. Blum[1]

> Full disclosure after an adverse event is the best policy. Patients want to know what happened, why it happened and that it will not happen again. Often, according to patient studies, this is the only reason they file a claim. If these concerns can be eased at the outset, it could save a lot of time, resources and psychological suffering for both patient and physician. Studies show that full disclosure does not lead to more litigation; in fact it has decreased the number of claims filed and the average amount of settlement. Plaintiffs' lawyers also seem to respect the policies, stating that they know better up front whether they have a legitimate claim.

> The move toward full disclosure by health-care institutions is only a recent trend, but it seems to be taking off. As more institutions establish full disclosure policies and more states enact legislation, which protect expressions of apology and sympathy accompanying those disclosures,

the result can only lead to a positive impact on improving patient care, treatment and the prevention of future errors.

— Jenny L. Pelt and Lynda Faldmo, "Physician Error and Disclosure"[2]

Lisa Shore and the Missing Corometric Machine[3]

Part 1: Missed Opportunities

On February 24, 2000, a coroner's jury comprised of three women and two men rendered an unprecedented verdict in the annals of Canadian health law. The jurors unanimously concluded that 10-year-old Lisa Shore had died between 6:20 a.m. and 7:00 a.m. on October 22, 1998, at the world-renowned Hospital for Sick Children (HSC) in Toronto, and that homicide was the means of death.

It is no understatement to say that the jury's verdict shook the venerable HSC to its core. HSC had unleashed a public relations disaster upon itself by virtue of the way it had behaved from October 22, 1998 (when Lisa died) until February 24, 2000 (the date of the homicide verdict). One would have thought that the homicide verdict would have provoked much more apologetic behaviour on the part of HSC. This would have been therapeutic for all. Unfortunately, HSC continued to support its nurses in the public eye and in their hearings at the College of Nurses, and it failed to ever proffer a meaningful, heartfelt apology to the Shores.

The devastating jury verdict triggered a cascade of negativity for the liable parties and the victims alike; it generated disciplinary proceedings before Ontario's College of Nurses for Lisa's two treating nurses and for HSC's Chief of Nursing; the two treating nurses were charged with criminal negligence causing death; Sharon Shore was delayed in her call to the Ontario Bar, and HSC was the recipient of reams of negative radio, television, print and internet publicity. This was adverse publicity which certainly damaged HSC's heretofore unblemished and well-earned reputation and no doubt had an impact on its recruitment and fundraising efforts. What then was the genesis of this unmitigated disaster for everyone involved, and what can be learned as a pedagogical exercise in terms of the possibility for apology to diminish the horrendous pain of a child's unanticipated death?

Lisa was born on November 20, 1987. She broke her right leg playing at the playground on February 11, 1998. Thereafter, she suffered excruciating pain in the injured leg. This pain was later diagnosed to be complex regional pain syndrome (CRPS), a non-life-threatening condition. Lisa was twice treated at Boston Children's Hospital, because the doctors at HSC thought her pain to be mostly psychosomatic.

Lisa's pain was so severe on October 21, 1998, that her mother, Sharon, brought her to the HSC emergency department. Lisa remained in the emergency department until 1:20 a.m. on October 22, 1998, at which time she was admitted to the orthopedic floor. Upon transfer, monitoring orders were entered in the hospital's "KIDCOM" computer system. It was at this point in the chain of events that the critical failure occurred: the nurses who were responsible for Lisa on the floor to which she was transferred failed to open or to access or to read these orders. Consequently, Lisa was not attached to an electronic monitor to measure her heart rate and respiratory rate. The deterioration in Lisa's vital signs which preceded her death was not responded to by the nurses, nor did the machine's alarms ever sound.

The two treating nurses reluctantly conceded through their lawyer at the inquest that if there was a monitor attached to Lisa (which Sharon Shore vehemently denied), then this monitor was not turned on and that's why the alarms didn't sound as Lisa's vital signs diminished, leading inexorably to her death. This agreement was announced to a packed coroner's court on January 17, 2000, by Ontario Deputy Chief Coroner T. James Cairns, MD, as follows:

> So for the purposes of the inquest, with that further evidence, with an analysis by a number of experts and with the agreement of all counsel, you can accept for the purposes of this inquest that if a monitor was in Lisa's room at 7 a.m., now it's up to you to decide later, but if a monitor was in Lisa's room at that time, then if it was in the room it either was not attached to Lisa and was turned off, or if it was attached to Lisa, it was turned off and the theory that was being put forth that electrical

activity from the heart, while not being productive electrical activity that would help her to have a heartbeat, may have in some way confused the monitor to think that she was alive when she wasn't alive, that is not an issue that needs to be addressed.

Everyone has accepted that if the monitor was in the room either attached or unattached to Lisa, it was in the off position and therefore that theory of the complex issues that were arising on the day that we stopped the inquest have now been addressed. I would just ask, Counsel, have I fairly represented the views that you all came to?

MR. GOMBERG: Yes, on behalf of the Shore family, I'm Frank Gomberg. I agree with that.

MR. HAWKINS: Yes, that's acceptable.

MR. KRKACHOVSKI: On behalf of G.E.M., yes, Mr. Coroner.

MS. POSNO: That's fine.

THE CORONER: I hope my Counsel isn't going to disagree with me.

MS. BROWN: No.

The two treating nurses later testified that Lisa had been attached to a monitor but the breathing part of the monitor was intentionally turned off by the more senior of the two nurses after three loud false alarms. In other words, rather than replacing the allegedly defective monitor, the senior nurse testified that she simply turned the breathing part of the monitor off. Neither Sharon Shore nor any of the other parents on the ward ever heard these three "phantom" alarms.

The coroner's jury clearly rejected the suggestion that these alarms had ever sounded. Even if the alarms had sounded, and in consequence the respiratory part of the monitor was turned off by the more senior nurse, the nurses and HSC had no explanation for why the cardiac component of the monitor never alarmed when Lisa's heart rate dropped. Their testimony was that they had not turned the cardiac component off, as it was mechanically impossible to do that. The obvious conclusion was that there was no monitor ever attached to Lisa and thus no alarms had ever sounded.

Rather than concede the fact that no monitor was ever used (which would have required a concomitant admission that the nursing care rendered to Lisa had been grossly negligent), HSC's lawyer called an HSC-employed biomedical engineer on November 9, 1999, to testify that the cardiac part of the monitor could be fooled into concluding that a child's stopped heart was still beating. If true, this would have been an explanation for why the cardiac part of the monitor never alarmed. This suggestion was made with no notice to the presiding coroner or to any of the participating lawyers. It led to a two-month adjournment of the inquest. Upon resuming the inquest, HSC recanted this ghost heartbeat suggestion by way of the January 17, 2000, agreement announced by Dr. Cairns and previously referred to. Instead of [offering] any apology up to and including the resumption of the inquest on January 17, 2000, HSC took a pummelling in court and in the press. This is how it played out in open court on November 9, 1999, leading to the adjournment until January 17, 2000, recantation.

THE CORONER: Mr. Gomberg?

MR. GOMBERG: Deputy Chief Coroner, I say this with the greatest of respect: this is outrageous. This is a theory that nobody has ever heard anything about. There are no expert reports that have been served on anyone, this is a Coroner's Inquest, so we have some latitude. To come up with the theory that nobody, including the Chief Coroner's Office, the Deputy Chief Coroner or the Crown Attorney, my friend Ms. Posno or I have heard anything about in the middle of a Coroner's Inquest, for an experienced litigation lawyer like my friend, is outrageous — he now calls a witness to give evidence that her heart, though it wasn't beating, was giving off some signals and that that explains why the Corometric, the heart part, didn't operate, is outrageous. This is the fourth or fifth inquest I've done in the last two years; I've never heard of anything like this. It is outrageous. We have written answers from the hospital to questions that were posed that say we don't know why that monitor didn't work. And, now, in the middle of the Coroner's Inquest, he comes up with a theory. It's outrageous. Those are my submissions.

The argument in open court, in the absence of the jury but in the presence of a dumbfounded media contingent (clearly hostile to HSC), continued:

MR. GOMBERG: Can I say something please? Mr. Hawkins, we're in a courtroom, and that doesn't mean that we're in Alice in Wonderland or in fantasy land. Mr. Hawkins has pulled a sleazy, cheap trick. Now, Mr. Hawkins is telling you things that are not true, because we had a meeting at the Hospital for Sick Children and had an opportunity to talk to the doctors, and I'm talking about Dr. Ro., who is the head of anesthesiology, I'm talking about Dr. Re., who is the head of nursing and I'm talking about the head of surgery, Dr. W., who as I understand it, is one of the chief doctors in the hospital. Not once did anybody ever say anything about this. Mr. Hawkins is not telling the truth.

MR. HAWKINS: I object most strongly to that.

MR. GOMBERG: You can object all you like.

MR. HAWKINS: Mr. B. has clearly indicated that he was first shown last Wednesday these wave forms. As of Friday, he ran these wave forms through the computer, and that's what he has produced here today.

MR. GOMBERG: Well, what are you talking about, meetings that we had?

Dr. Cairns summarized the situation much more succinctly:

We can argue this issue appropriately with proper production of material in advance, but I don't see how we can possibly pursue this particular item with this particular witness at this particular time, since we have had no production. I would want this reduced to writing and I would want to be able to get independent experts to review this, if that is a line that you're intending to take along. I must say, I, personally, unless you've got a different explanation, I consider this an *ambush* of the process [author's emphasis].

The two-month adjournment (November 12, 1999 – January 17, 2000) would not have been necessary had this ghost heartbeat construct not been concocted. HSC could have avoided the following headlines in the local and national newspapers:

"Confusion Delays Inquest"

"Lawyer Calls Testimony 'Outrageous'"

"Status of Cardiac Monitor at Question in Girl's Death"

"Girl's Death Not Due to Monitor, Lawyer Says"

"Hospital Covering for Nurses: Mother"

"Coroner Fumes Over Ambush"

When it dropped the "ghost heartbeats" theory on January 17, 2000, HSC was reeling from its self-inflicted wounds. It is easy to infer that the jurors were unimpressed. On February 3, 2000, juror L.D., on the pretext of asking a question of clarification of a nursing educator who was testifying (which inquest jurors are permitted to do), asked the following:

BY JUROR 4
Q. The testimony that we've heard by the nurses telling us what was done, what we find wasn't done —
A. Mm-hmm.

Q. — filling in flow sheets with parts of what should have been filled in, we've heard of instances supposedly where people have lied to one another, improper forms being made or errors being made in certain documents. And I'm sure, Dr., if I'm allowed to ask this but to me this sounds like a cover-up.

A. I mean, I —

Q. We've been given a smokescreen.

A. Mm-hmm.

Q. Now, I'm not asking you to answer it, but my thought is —

THE CORONER: I don't think this witness, in her capacity, is able to answer that question.

BY JUROR 4

Q. I do have one other comment. I realize Sick Children's Hospital is well known and unblemished, basically, and I hope that this situation is just an isolated case and it covers the whole iceberg and not just the tip. A. I assure you this has been unlike anything I've ever experienced in my career. If that gives you any assurance or reassurance, it's been extremely distressing for all of us and unusual, never seen it before, unheard of, distressing, extremely tragic, extremely unfortunate. I wish we could all roll back the hands of time and fix something to prevent this.

Unfortunately for HSC, the front page of the next day's newspaper added water to an already floundering ship. The headline screamed "Sick Kids Cover-Up Charged: Inquest Juror Points Finger at Toronto Hospital." Where was the apology? It seemed that the apology was lost in cyberspace — just as the KIDCOM orders had been lost in cyberspace.

When it seemed that things couldn't possibly get worse for HSC, they did. An audiotape describing the conditions of all patients on the ward, including Lisa, was erased and consequently never furnished to the coroner. The missing emergency orders were not located by HSC management until January 26, 1999 (because the administration couldn't figure out how to retrieve the orders from the computer system), even though one of the nurses had printed them up on October 27, 1999 (five days after Lisa's death), and retained them until she brought them to court at my request on January 28, 2000. She apparently succeeded in locating the orders in the computer system, whereas the HSC administration including its computer experts had failed in its search.

On January 27, 2000, all of these calamitous revelations were compounded even further: observations by the jurors led them to believe that at least one of the nurses in the body of the courtroom was signalling answers to one of the two culpable nurses as she testified:

> THE CORONER: Just before we begin again, at the break the Coroner's Constable has brought to my attention that the jury have indicated to the Coroner's Constable that they have concerns that this witness, while answering questions, that it appears to them that certain members of the audience, and it's their impression, is assisting the witness with answers by certain body movements.
>
> I would remind the audience that this witness is on the witness stand, and even the appearance of prompting an answer is inappropriate. And if it continues, I will have to do something about it. The indication through the Coroner's Constable is that before the witness answers a question, it is the jury's impression that there is nodding of heads or shaking of heads before the answer is given.
>
> That is entirely inappropriate if it's going on. Whether it's being done intentionally or not, I am not in a position to say, but it's inappropriate and I would like to see it cease immediately, otherwise other steps will be taken.

This was an anathema to the position of HSC — because if the jury thinks something is happening, then it's happening. It hardly improved matters that both the *Globe and Mail* and the *Toronto Star* on January 28, 2000, each cited the concern of the jurors that a negligent nurse was being coached while testifying under oath.

The final indignity to HSC consisted of the already mentioned devastating post-verdict editorials harshly condemning the hospital.

The titles to the editorials were ominous: "Hospital Homicide," "Lisa Shore Didn't Have to Die" and "Sick Kids Mistreats Grieving Parents."

What then could have obviated most, if not all, of these cataclysmic events? I submit that a proper apology was necessary, but one was never offered. A visually simple chronology of events highlights when apologetic intervention would likely have achieved a desirable goal. It was surprising and disappointing that with all of the administrative, public relations, medical, technological and intellectual brainpower at HSC, the apologetic comments that were eventually proffered were too contrived and too deficient to constitute anything more than non-apologies or pseudo-apologies (for reasons to be discussed later in this paper) and consequently served only to insult the surviving family members.

October 22, 1998: Lisa's death at HSC

September 30, 1999: Civil case settled before mediator, retired Court of Appeal Justice W. D. Griffiths

November 8, 1999: Coroner's Inquest begins

November 12, 1999: Coroner's Inquest adjourns over "ghost heartbeats"

January 17, 2000: Coroner's Inquest resumes when HSC abandons "ghost heartbeats" position

February 24, 2000: Coroner's Inquest verdict rocks HSC

It is noteworthy that the civil litigation had been settled at mediation in order to obviate any suggestion that the Shores' quest for answers and for justice was monetarily motivated. As such, apology was certainly available to HSC between Lisa's death on October 22, 1998, and the mediation; at the mediation on September 30, 1999;

or during the Inquest (November 8, 1999 – February 24, 2000). Indeed, the lengthy adjournment, because of the suggestion of ghost heartbeats, presented an excellent opportunity for apology: the tort damages had already been paid, HSC knew it was going to abandon the ghost heartbeats strategy upon resumption of the inquest, and an apology would have been inadmissible at the inquest. There was no apparent legal or factual reason that no apology was forthcoming at that time. The only apology ever made to the Shores up to the conclusion of the inquest was delivered by Dr. J. Re., Chief of Nursing, from the witness box on February 8, 2000. This is what Dr. Re. said when questioned by her lawyer:

> Q. I understand, Dr. Re., that there is something you would like to say on behalf of the Hospital to the family.
> A. I would. Mr. and Mrs. Shore and your family members, I have sat here throughout the inquest, we've met on two previous occasions and on behalf of our institution, let me say how terribly sorry we all are, because we failed you as an institution. We are terribly sorry.

This apology was delivered in an emotionless, impersonal way, in a sterile courtroom in downtown Toronto. I have [a copy of] the actual audio of this apology in the late Dr. Re.'s voice [and] the transcript doesn't reflect her lack of emotion. Dr. Re. was present at the September 30, 1999, mediation with her lawyer and a Healthcare Insurance Reciprocal of Canada (HIROC) representative. No one from the medical or nursing staffs or from the HSC administration attended the mediation. No apology was offered at mediation. Opportunity missed.

After this pseudo-, non-apology by Dr. Re. from the witness box on February 8, 2000, the next pseudo-, non-apology was offered by Dr. Alan Goldbloom, HSC senior vice-president, at HSC's post-inquest press conference on February 24, 2000. Significantly, the Shores were not invited to this event. The following are excerpts from this oral apology:

We are deeply saddened by the tragedy of Lisa Shore's death. Clearly the Hospital for Sick Children failed Lisa Shore and failed the Shore family. We will live with this forever. We are profoundly sorry for what has happened. We are determined to do everything humanly possible to ensure that such a tragedy never happens again. [. . .]

Finally, I want to say to the members of the Shore family that no words could possibly express how sorry and devastated all of us are by this tragedy. The people who devote their careers to this institution are here to help children and to support families. When we fail to do that it is devastating for all of us. We offer them our deepest sympathies. We apologize for the mistakes that have been made. We are terribly sorry. We will all live with this forever. [. . .]

Our apology and our regret over this tragic death are very sincere. I understand how the Shore family must feel. I understand their anger. They have suffered a loss that is unspeakable. Their grief must be unspeakable. Nothing can change what happened. We continue to offer our apologies and we continue to feel in this hospital that we have let the family down.

Two additional truncated and remarkably similar (no doubt coordinated) non-apologies had been previously delivered as follows: "This was a very sad event and we offer sincere condolences to the entire Shore family," and "Lisa's death is a very sad thing. The hospital offers its sincere condolences to the entire Shore family."

A further non-apology was issued by Michael Strofolino, president and CEO of HSC, in a press release on March 6, 2000, dealing with the nurses reporting themselves to the Ontario College of Nurses. As Mr. Strofolino put it, "We apologize again to the Shore family for the pain we have caused them. They can be sure that the College will review the nursing issues in detail."

By issuing this apology to the press, Strofolino gave the impression of being less concerned about the family than he was about the public perception of HSC. In retrospect, it is clear that this apology was merely an attempt to avoid the further adverse publicity which was about to be unleashed upon the nurses and HSC by Sharon

Shore's imminent formal letters of complaint to the Ontario College of Nurses.

The final purported apology occurred at my law office on March 7, 2000. Michael Strofolino, Sharon and Bill Shore and I were the only ones present. In this further deficient apology, Strofolino refused to accede to the Shores' request that HSC fire the two culprit nurses — an act which was critical as part of reparation and promise to reform; acknowledging the offence and effecting reparation; showing remorse, making restitution and foregoing repetition; repudiation of bad behaviour (bad actors); promise to behave correctly in the future and atonement and compensation; and the corroboration of factual blame, acceptance of blame, identification of harm, and reform and redress. Indeed, Strofolino's demeanour was defiant, and although some of what he said was intended to be conciliatory, the message was that HSC's non-cooperation wasn't really its fault, because initially the death was a coroner's case and more recently the nurses were involved in disciplinary proceedings. This refusal to take responsibility flies in the face of all apology theories and ignores the reality that the inquest coroner, the inquest jury, the media and any other fair-minded courtroom observers had concluded that the nursing care rendered to Lisa was abysmally deficient and the HSC investigation to determine what had happened was equally deficient. Opportunity lost.

Part 2: Ethical Emergencies

Philip C. Hébert MD, Ph.D., an internationally recognized bio-ethics educator and author, was before his recent retirement a family physician at Sunnybrook Health Sciences Centre. He is Professor Emeritus of Family Medicine at the University of Toronto. He chairs the Research Ethics Board and acts as a bioethics consultant for the hospital.

I asked Dr. Hébert why doctors are bad at apology and explanation when unexpected death occurs. His answer in part was:

> Doctors are perfectionists. They don't like acknowledging their fallibility. To do so is like swallowing a watermelon whole — it sticks in your throat.

Dr. Hébert offered how HSC ought to have dealt with the Shore family. He unhesitatingly and forcefully articulated the following:

> HSC ought to have met with the family straight away. I don't know why that did not happen. Lisa's death was the ethical equivalent of a medical emergency. There are few ethical emergencies in medicine. This was one of them. Lying about mistakes as was done in the Shore matter is almost as bad as the actual mistakes. In Shore, HSC was not prepared in a systemic way to deal with error. Perhaps, the hospital didn't know how to analyze error or to determine culpability. There was an inability to tie together the loose ends at the end of their analysis. But lying about what transpired is antithetical to everything medicine and nursing stand for.

I asked Dr. Hébert to define an ethical emergency. He responded:

> Ethical emergencies are those situations where there is the potential for a complete loss of trust in the health-care professionals and the health-care institutions by the survivors. The longer the failure to explain and apologize continues, the greater the chasm between the survivors and the professionals. This situation pertains in all unexpected death scenarios whether or not the deaths were preventable.

Dr. Hébert reviewed each of the three cases in our trilogy. [Gomberg's complete research paper discusses three cases.] He felt that each precipitated an ethical emergency.

> Doctors often respond to bad outcomes in a cavalier way — "that death can occur." However, it is vitally important that the health-care professionals appropriately handle the unexpected nature of outcomes like death. What is being done to understand these unexpected outcomes? The more serious the outcome, the more seriously the health-care institution should take the case. The family doesn't want to see the hospital proceeding as if it's "business as usual." Adopting the "these things happen" approach is not the way to respond. These are not pure accidents such as if someone gets hit by a meteorite.

Dr. Hébert concurred that in the Shore case:

1. Lisa wasn't sick;
2. They gave her morphine;
3. This created a dangerous milieu;
4. Lisa required professional monitoring;
5. Lisa didn't get professional monitoring;
6. A medical emergency ensued;
7. The medical emergency wasn't appropriately responded to;
8. Lisa died;
9. This created an ethical emergency.

When ethical emergencies like this arise, Dr. Hébert said that what must be done to be effective is to advise the family right away what is known and what is unknown. Ongoing communication with the family is critical, and that communication must be a dialogue which allows for questions. If answers are unavailable, they should be sought and provided as they become available. Transparency is critical.

Dr. Hébert explained that the Shore case got off track when the hospital personnel failed to meet with the Shores to tell them what was known in the immediate aftermath of Lisa's death. The "whole process got derailed." Where there was chaos, the hospital ought to have attempted to impose some order. It failed to do that.

When I asked Dr. Hébert about the hospital's inability to locate the missing orders which Lisa's nurse printed up a few days after Lisa's death; the failure to segregate the Corometric monitor; the erasure of the tape; the "ghost heartbeats"; and the nurses signalling answers to the witness at coroner's court, Dr. Hébert called all of this:

> a litany of cover-up. It's egregiously unprofessional. It doesn't work. They wanted an outcome they couldn't manufacture. They couldn't do it because the coroner's jury had oversight over this series of events. It's a failure of the medical and health-care systems when legal oversight must be brought into it. These are moral and medical emergencies and must be handled within the health-care system. That's what professional

training is all about. The real professional says, "I'm responsible. I made a mistake. The buck stops with me." They say it regardless of any consequences, legal, moral or monetary. If a health-care professional makes a mistake, he or she shouldn't compound it by lying about it.

Part 3: Too Little, Not Too Late

I asked Sharon Shore what kind of apology she wanted from HSC. This is what she wrote on March 1, 2011, more than 12 years after Lisa's death:

> My daughter is dead. I blame you — you, the two nurses who were supposed to be caring for her but instead left her to die and then tried to cover it up, and you, the hospital who helped them cover it up and who continues to protect and defend them to this day. You, the two nurses, you never apologized at all, directly or indirectly. Even when you were found to have committed professional misconduct by the College of Nurses, you still did not express an iota of remorse. Why should you, when the hospital that employed you — and still employs you, as far as I know — has wrapped you in its protective cocoon and denied that you did anything wrong? I suppose I should give you a modicum of credit for being honest about your lack of remorse, considering that you lied about everything else.
>
> You, the hospital, you knew what happened was not "system error" — a convenient little catchphrase used to excuse anything that takes place in a hospital setting, no matter how egregious or criminal. You tried to say it was, and you still say it, but you couldn't fool the lay people who made up the coroner's jury, who found my daughter's death a homicide. The jury was not any smarter or less smart than you, only more honest.
>
> I have been asked to write about the apology I would have liked to receive. That apology would have three things which yours did not: it would have been timely, it would have acknowledged that the two nurses had been grossly negligent, and the two nurses would have been fired and reported to the College of Nurses for professional misconduct.
>
> No apology in the world could ever have assuaged my pain, but

a genuine one from you would have allowed me to forgive. Instead, your apologies were nothing but hot air. Each one made me hate you a little more.

You, the hospital, employer of the nurses, you did apologize on several occasions. The first apology came at the end of the coroner's inquest, a year and a half after my daughter's death, by your chief of nursing. We had met several times before, and we both attended each day of the weeks-long inquest. How could you fail to realize that your nursing chief's rehearsed, emotionally flat apology proffered from the witness stand at the eleventh hour to the gathered media and hospital executives would be seen as offensive and insincere? Your second apology, by your vice-president at the press conference following the inquest, was solely for the media's benefit since we weren't there to hear it. How was that sincere and meaningful? You put a bit more effort into your third apology, by having your president apologize to me privately. But did you really think that these words, coming as they did from this gold-jewellery-laden man in his expensive suit, and without any more substance than the first two apologies, would mean anything more than those others did? I said to your president that his apology was worthless unless he did something about the two nurses — fire them, I said — and he refused. You fired your chief of nursing instead, making her the scapegoat for your sins. Was that supposed to appease me?

Then there is the letter from the president that contained a promise that you broke soon after. Not only did you make empty apologies and refuse to take any real action, you outright lied to me — in writing. Is it really a surprise that I have nothing but contempt for you?

I accept that you didn't apologize to me in the days and even weeks following my daughter's death. You didn't know exactly what had happened, and the coroner's office was involved. But there was a point relatively soon after when you did know — and you knew beyond a reasonable doubt, as the lawyers say, that your nurses had been grossly negligent.

As a mother, I can say to you that this was the time to make the first apology — along with a commitment that when the dust settled, you would take appropriate action to deal with these nurses. As a lawyer, I understand the reasons that might have prevented you from saying anything that soon. But there was nothing to stop you from taking action behind the scenes. How much more believable an apology would have been when eventually tendered, if it was accompanied by hard evidence that the issues had already been appropriately dealt with.

Your apologies, without acknowledgment and ownership of wrongdoing, were glib and self-serving. I needed you to acknowledge that your nurses had been grossly negligent. I needed to hear you say that what happened — my daughter's death — should not have happened.

Part of an admission of wrongdoing is taking responsibility for it. You did not. Along with responsibility, there should be remorse, shame, guilt — emotion! — that this happened under your watch. There was none of that.

Most of all, I needed to see concrete action taken, proof that you would not — could not — employ nurses who did not follow hospital policies, procedures, or doctor's orders, and who lied to cover up their wrongdoings.

It is still not too late. I am here.

Open Arms

Open Arms Patient Advocacy Society, founded by Rick and Rose Lundy of Calgary, is a non-profit society committed to providing assistance and support to patients and their families who have experienced adverse medical events. Much of the society's work is focused on helping people find answers to questions associated with their particular situations. These endeavours often lead to changes which improve the quality and delivery of health care for everyone.

The story of Open Arms began on a July evening in 2006 when Rose began to bleed from what initially appeared to be an uncomplicated miscarriage. She was three and a half months pregnant at the time. Rick took Rose to the Peter Lougheed Centre of the Calgary General Hospital where she began to hemorrhage in the overcrowded emergency room.

In the next three hours, Rick joined the long line to see the triage nurse five times. "I kept going up and the nurse kept telling me there was nothing they could do, because there were no beds," Rick said. In the meantime, fetal tissue was dropping out of Rose's shorts and blood was running down her legs to pool on the floor. "It was so humiliating," Rose recalled. Horrified, many of the other 40 people in the ER waiting area kept saying, "You need help."

Rick rushed between Rose and lining up yet again to see the triage nurse. "She kept getting weaker. Nobody would come out to check on her. I felt so helpless," Rick said. Finally, there was a shift change and the new triage nurse told Rick to "bring her up." But by this time Rose was too weak to walk.

With the help of a lady on crutches from knee surgery, Rick managed to get Rose into a wheelchair. Immediately upon seeing Rose, the triage nurse called a special alert code. Rose, who had started to convulse, was soon receiving the medical attention she had been needing for several hours.

Rose recalled the doctors and nurses saying, "We're so sorry, we're so sorry."

"I sensed they wanted to say more, but couldn't," Rose said. Meanwhile, Rick kept asking the doctors and nurses, "How could this happen? How can someone bleed all over the floor for so long in this country and be ignored?"

After leaving the hospital, Rose went into a deep depression. "It was the humiliation and helplessness, not the miscarriage itself," said Rose. She had previously had a miscarriage before the birth of their five-year-old twin boys. Rick was also deeply affected and required treatment for post-traumatic stress.

In the depths of their personal suffering, Rick and Rose asked each other, "What are we going to do to help others?" A week after the night in the ER, Rick made a phone call that started a media frenzy across the country. A Global news van was parked in front of their house for so long that a new neighbour thought Rick worked for Global. The *Calgary Herald* ranked the Lundys' experience the top news story of 2006.

Within days, Rick and Rose became the face of health-care mishaps in Canada. People kept calling the Lundy home wanting to share their experiences and asking for advice. When the couple could not find an advocacy group that they could recommend to callers, they decided to form one themselves.

Recognition of their role in helping others brought healing and closure to Rose and Rick. "At first I felt like I wanted to replace the lost baby. Then I accepted how blessed I was to have had two boys at once. I understood the purpose of the miscarriage was for me to help other people," Rose said.

Open Arms quickly grew out of the Lundys' continuing assistance to others. The group was started in March 2007, only months after Rose's miscarriage, and it was granted non-profit status a year later. "The people we needed just appeared and they keep appearing," Rose said.

Today, a diverse group of volunteers is led by a board that includes a policy analyst, a media/electronic technical expert, a number of physicians including a psychiatrist, medical malpractice lawyers, a former Alberta Health executive and, of course, individuals with personal experience of adverse events, such as Tiana Melnyk.

A Calgary teacher and community volunteer, Tiana joined the Open Arms board as part of her goal to provide a voice to individuals who are under-represented in health care. At 17, she was diagnosed with rheumatoid arthritis and has experienced first-hand the consequences of a system which sometimes lacks the resources to provide adequate help to individuals with chronic illnesses.

As chairperson, Rick brings considerable business expertise to the board. A 1990 graduate of the Southern Alberta Institute of Technology in business administration, he manages the Inglewood Golf and Curling Club in Calgary and has served on the boards of restaurant and tourism associations. Rose, who has a background in biological and environmental sciences, is the secretary for Open Arms. She also helps to raise funds for the society.

Rick estimates that he has received close to 400 telephone calls and emails from people who want to tell their stories and receive general guidance. An additional 200 have become clients of Open Arms, which means the Lundys or specially trained advocates have helped them in a variety of ways. Approximately 30 percent of the clients have had family members die as the result of medical errors.

Open Arms has been involved with a wide array of cases occurring in many different settings. Most clients live in Alberta; however, Open Arms has dealt and continues to deal with people from all parts of Canada. "Our medical system usually does an excellent job. But when things go wrong, we've become the go-to people. We see the worst of the worst," Rick said.

Advocates from Open Arms help clients prepare for meetings with representatives from health regions and attend the meetings with them. Clients often tell Rick they couldn't have gone without him. Rick and his team assist clients in understanding all available options from groups such as colleges of physicians and surgeons, nurses' associations, provincial ombudsmen, the media and legal professionals. They will also attend doctors' appointments with clients.

Open Arms assisted Marlene Kovacs, who had a colonoscopy in the fall of 2007 before returning to her job as a teacher in Calgary. During the procedure, which revealed nothing of concern, Kovacs' spleen was ruptured. Sent home to rest, she soon realized something was terribly wrong and returned to hospital by ambulance where she waited in the ER for six hours. It took another eight hours to diagnose internal bleeding and a ruptured spleen. She was already in kidney failure by the time she received five blood transfusions and her spleen was removed. Today, she is on dialysis waiting for a kidney transplant. "My advocate, Rick Lundy, was the only one who understood my difficulties. He gave me the tools to stand up for my rights and fight back. When I finally met with the Health Region, they admitted my care was not ideal and they made changes to the system so this does not happen to anybody else. Open Arms saved my life and gave me back some human dignity where I felt it had been taken away."

Darlene Durand of Calgary received help from Open Arms in obtaining answers to questions related to a misdiagnosis.

> My story began when I was diagnosed with thyroid cancer. Trusting my doctor's findings, I decided to have the thyroid removed, but once it was, I was told that they had found no cancer. They had misdiagnosed my condition and then basically sent me on my way after breaking the news. I began to wonder how this could have happened and tried to get answers. This process was frustrating and stressful, because I was getting nowhere with the medical system.
>
> Then a friend told me about Open Arms and I contacted them. Rick

Lundy immediately helped me feel at ease and confident that I could get the answers I needed. He provided me with information on how to work within the medical system to finally get a meeting scheduled with the Health Region. Going into the meeting, my family and I hoped for honesty and transparency. Members of the Health Region did give answers to the best of their ability and this provided closure for us.

The most important thing I learned through this experience is that you are in charge of your own health. You as the patient have every right to question a diagnosis and ask for a second opinion.

Currently, Open Arms is helping a woman find answers as to how her severely depressed husband could have hanged himself from a gurney using a transfer belt while in hospital. "This lady, like all of our clients, wants two things. She wants to know what happened and what changes are being made so it won't happen again," Rick said.

"We're effective because we're in the trenches with the people. We know what they're going through," said Rose.

Rick knows "the ropes" of how to get things done. "I've come to learn how it all works and comes together," Rick said.

In addition to supporting and assisting families, Open Arms is active in liaising with the health-care community to bring systematic changes to the Alberta health-care system. In the months following Rose's miscarriage, she and Rick were asked to participate in a patient-care advisory committee. More recently, they were invited to provide input into the amending of the Alberta Health Information Act and to set up health-service groups. The couple meet regularly with politicians and health-services executives and continue to speak out on issues related to patient safety.

In early 2010, Rick told the *Calgary Herald* that the refusal of the Alberta Health Services to release the full report by the Health Quality Council of Alberta on four serious mistakes at Alberta Children's Hospital undermined public confidence. Rick and other patient advocates argued that it is difficult to restore public trust without full disclosure of medical errors. "When patients go through something, they are looking for transparency and honesty," he said.

"When an investigation is done, it's not about pointing the finger or blaming anybody. It's to find out the facts and makes changes so it doesn't happen to somebody else."

The Lundys understand that their effectiveness is dependent on having good relations with everyone — health-care providers and health systems, politicians, the media and clients. "We work in a respectful manner without attacking," said Rose.

She and Rick feel a sense of accomplishment when clients say how much Open Arms has helped them to heal and that they can now shut that door and move on. Another source of satisfaction is the changes made by the Calgary Health Region following Rose's ordeal. The time social workers are available in emergency rooms has been doubled from eight to 16 hours a day to help families dealing with various emotional issues, including miscarriage.

The health region also established special privacy rooms designed for miscarrying women. Such rooms were recommended shortly after the Lundys' experience in July 2006 and instituted three months later after two other women had miscarriages in front of strangers in a crowded emergency room. "Many of the women who use the rooms have called to thank us," Rick said.

Not people to rest on past achievements, the Lundys and their team are planning to have trained volunteer advocates in Alberta's half-dozen largest cities and in the north.

As well, Open Arms will be launching a program on mental illness, especially focusing on the associated stigma. They will be investigating the sparse resources allocated to mental health and will make recommendations to the provincial government and health services on how to improve care of mentally ill Albertans. "One in five people in this country suffer from some form of mental illness. It is so important and yet the stigma associated with mental illness is still strong," Rick said. "When was the last time you saw a fundraiser for depression or anxiety like you do for cancer or heart disease?"

Over the years, the Lundys have had their share of obstacles and disappointments along with successes. They have encountered individuals who are resistant to change or unwilling to accept responsibility, and experienced frustrations related to the complexity of government and health-care systems. Regardless, the Lundys and their team at Open Arms persist. "When I see someone take out a picture of a loved one they've lost because of an error and know I can help — that's what keeps me going," Rick said.

The Spark

The length of a life is not necessarily indicative of its significance. Born on June 14, 1999, Carter Tapp was the second child of Darren and Sharon Tapp and known as their little "Twinkle." Carter strangled to death on his IV tubing in an Edmonton hospital 35 days before his first birthday. His death was the spark that initiated many improvements in pediatric care throughout Canada and elsewhere. This is the story of some of these achievements.

Last Days of Carter's Life

On the morning of May 7, 2000, Sharon took Carter to the local health centre. He was diagnosed with pneumonia and was given oxygen through nasal cannula and treatment to ease his breathing. An intravenous line for fluids and antibiotics was inserted into a vein in his hand. Carter was then transferred to the pediatric ward at the hospital.

Sharon spent the day with Carter. At one point, when he had fallen asleep, she left the room to phone Darren with an update on their son's condition. A few minutes later, when Sharon entered Carter's room, she noticed he had rolled in bed and the IV tubing had draped around his body. Recalling that day, Sharon said, "I spoke to two different nurses that day, Carter's primary day-shift nurse and primary night-shift nurse, about this worrisome situation. They both told me this was not a concern. Tragically, I believed them."

Carter responded well to treatment. By late in the morning of the following day, May 8, he no longer required oxygen support, and the amount of fluids he was receiving through the IV was reduced to just enough to keep the vein open for periodic doses of antibiotics, a common practice to reduce the number of invasive procedures. Darren and Sharon were told that, if all continued to go well, their son would be released from hospital the next day, May 9.

At midday, Sharon received a call from the daycare centre telling her that Kyra, Carter's three-year-old sister, was starting to run a fever. Sharon left Carter to take Kyra to the doctor and, after the appointment, she returned to Carter's room with Kyra. In late afternoon, Sharon left to take Kyra home to stay with Darren. She was planning to return to the hospital, stay overnight and bring Carter home the following morning. Before leaving, Sharon told Carter's primary-care nurse about her plans.

In less than an hour, the pediatrician phoned the Tapp home to tell them Carter was in cardiac arrest and they were trying to resuscitate him. He had been found in his crib without a pulse and was not breathing. The pediatrician said he did not know what happened, but he did not think it had anything to do with Carter's pneumonia. As Darren and Sharon were preparing to leave and making arrangements for Kyra's care, the pediatrician phoned again to say Carter had been resuscitated and was going to be transferred to the university hospital.

When the Tapps arrived at Carter's room, the resuscitation team was still at work and the transport team was standing by to take him to the university hospital.

The pediatrician took Darren and Sharon into another room where he told them he still didn't know what had happened. Sharon asked him to find out if the IV tubing had been wrapped around Carter's neck. Months later, at the fatality inquiry, the pediatrician said Sharon's question was the first he had heard of the Tapps' concerns over Carter becoming wrapped in the lines.

On May 8, Carter's primary-care nurse told the pediatrician that the IV tube had been wrapped around Carter's neck but not tightly, because she could get a finger between the tube and his neck. Later, it was revealed that the tube had been wrapped three times around Carter's neck. The pediatrician speculated that the tube wasn't tight when the nurse examined Carter, because the crib rail had been dropped reducing tension on the tube.

After Carter was taken to the university hospital, Sharon went to speak with his primary-care nurse. She found the nurse cleaning the room and noticed that almost everything had been put into the trash, including the IV. When requested by Sharon, the nurse retrieved it from the garbage in a room across the hall.

At the time, Sharon did not think to request the video security tapes from which it would have been determined how often a nurse or a respiratory therapist had checked on Carter. By the time she and Darren asked to see the tapes, they had been reused.

When the Tapps arrived at the pediatric intensive care unit at the university hospital, they found Carter on a ventilator and in a deep coma. Red and purple marks were visible around his neck. Sharon requested that a record be made of the marks on Carter's chart.

Carter was given many tests and all confirmed severe brain damage. After waiting two days in order to give Carter every chance, the Tapps made the hardest decision of their lives. Carter died in his parents' arms shortly after being removed from the ventilator.

The Years Following

Shortly after Carter's death, an autopsy was performed which confirmed that he died from lack of oxygen as a result of the IV tubing around his neck. The autopsy report was sent to the Fatality Review Board. In due course, a Public Fatality Inquiry was called. Such an inquiry is similar in intent to a coroner's inquest in other provinces; it is concerned with finding fact, not fault. At an inquiry, a Crown attorney presents the information to a provincial court judge, who can make non-binding recommendations to help prevent similar tragedies from occurring in the future. Other interested parties, for example, the lawyer acting on behalf of the deceased's family, and lawyers representing the hospital and doctors, can also ask questions. The fatality inquiry started in February 2001 and was completed in September of the same year. The report was released in August 2002.

Between Carter's death and the release of the fatality inquiry report, Carter's parents, health authorities and others worked in various ways to prevent the death of children under similar circumstances. Darren and Sharon appeared on national and local radio and television programs and participated in interviews for Alberta newspapers. As well, the Canadian Press wire service made their story available to newspapers across the country. They contributed the story of Carter's death to the book *Medical Nightmares: The Human Face of Errors*.

Sharon contacted the Children's Safety Association of Canada (safekid.org), which reviewed the circumstances surrounding Carter's death. In addition, Carter's case was entered into the United States Food and Drug Administration Manufacturer and User Facility Device Experience Database. The Tapps established the website twinkle.ca.

In early February 2001, Sharon and Darren wrote to the Alberta Minister of Health and to the federal Minister of Health. The Alberta minister said he would direct all of the regional health authorities to implement any recommendations that the inquiry judge made. The federal minister offered to assist in the development and distribution of relevant information.

Also in early February 2001, the Tapps sent press releases to the media. The releases included a brief synopsis of what had happened to Carter, information on other fatal and near-fatal cases of children strangling on IV and oxygen tubes and their suggested recommendations. In particular, the Tapps thought the length of IV tubing used with infants should be decreased and the method of delivery should be changed from the current pole pump to a syringe pump kept in a fanny pack. They also felt there should be some form of adult supervision at all times and an IV needs-versus-risk assessment should be made in each case.

The Tapps wrote to Health Canada, as did health-care officials and physicians. In July 2002, Health Canada issued a notice to hospitals that outlined a number of guidelines to increase the safe use of IV tubing and monitor leads. In response to concerns raised by health-care providers across the country regarding the ability to carry out these recommendations, a Patient Safety Workshop was organized by Health Canada and the Canadian Association of Paediatric Care Centres and held on June 14, 2003, in Calgary. At this workshop, improvements were made to the initial Health Canada recommendations.

In 2008, the British Columbia Institute of Technology (BCIT) announced the invention of the IV Infant Safety Vest. The work was done under a contract from the BC Children's Hospital.

Subsequently, BCIT researchers had three of their inventions evaluated by nurses. The IV Infant Safety Vest was selected for further development and evaluation in actual clinical use. Made of light-weight material, the vest fits snugly around the child's upper body. It gathers all lines and tubing from the upper body in a special sleeve incorporated into the vest and channels them to the lower part of the body, where they emerge and are then hooked up to various pieces of equipment. Designed for patients six to 36 months of age, the vest is disposable and can handle multiple lines. At the time of this writing, patent applications had been made in more than six countries. "Once we have the idea protected, we can talk to potential manufacturers with confidence," said Thom Bellaire, research analyst at BCIT and member of the vest development team.

Not long after Carter's death, Capital Health introduced policies to minimize the risk of IV tube strangulation. In December 2000, nurses were provided with devices allowing IV tubes to be detached when not in use. Later, nurses were ordered to do risk assessments of infants likely to become tangled, keep records of any incidents and increase monitoring. As well, mechanical methods to reduce risk of entanglement were sought and collaboration was established with Bill Reilly, inventor of the IV Medical Line Stabilizer (ivydevices.ca).

Reilly, who holds a bachelor's degree in public health, was employed by a construction company that was working at the hospital at the time of Carter's death. Reilly was responsible for industrial hygiene and for minimizing the impact of construction on hospital activities. News of the tragic event spread quickly, including to employees of the construction company. "It just came to me if you put a sleeve over the IV line that would keep the line away from the child," Reilly said.

He presented preliminary drawings to health authorities, who liked the concept and asked Reilly to have a model made. The result was the IV stabilizer, which is a two-foot long channel, slightly larger in diameter than typical IV tubing, made from food-grade plastic. The stabilizer is flexible enough to allow larger IV and other tubing within its channel, yet rigid enough to protect patients from accidental entanglement with IV tubing. The IV stabilizer is suitable for patients six to 18 months in age.

An extensive clinical trial was conducted to determine the effectiveness and ensure the safety of the stabilizer. The device is still being used in Capital Health hospitals, occasionally in hospitals outside of Alberta and in home-care settings. "The stabilizer has been successful. There hasn't been an incident associated with its use in 10 years," Reilly said.

Reilly holds patents in both Canada and the United States on his invention, but has been unable to interest a large manufacturer because of low financial return. To date, he has sold approximately 20,000 stabilizers. They are made in Edmonton and shipped to his home in Grand Prairie, and he supplies them to hospitals as requested. Reilly makes just enough money to pay for production and related business expenses, and the required insurance. "I'm willing to continue as long as the stabilizers are useful," he said.

During the fatality inquiry, Judge Shelagh Creagh heard nurses and physicians say repeatedly they had never known or heard of IV tubing being a strangulation risk until Carter's death. Although there had been no reports in the medical literature of risks associated with the use of IV tubing for infants, a few accounts of fatal and near-fatal strangulations had been reported in the popular press and government databases. Two years after the fatality inquiry, the international medical community was alerted to the risks by the paper, "Strangulation with Intravenous Tubing: A Previously Undescribed Adverse Advent in Children."[1] Fatalities of children by strangulation on loose wires and cords, such as drapery cords and pacifier cords, were well documented at the time.

Robert Kain, father of a baby girl in Carter's room, testified that tubes were around his neck on two occasions and a nurse spoke of Carter in a disrespectful manner. Both allegations were denied by nurses. Unhappy with the attention their daughter was receiving, Kain and his wife took her home an hour before Carter's death, despite their pediatrician's request that she stay an extra day for observation.

The Tapp family lawyer, Eleanor Olszewski, submitted more than 20 recommendations to the judge. She also told Creagh that hospitals must educate staff to listen to patients' families. "Mrs. Tapp was concerned about the tangling issue. The Kains were concerned about the tangling issue," Olszewski said.

"The fact these systems pose a danger to infants is, in hindsight, obvious and . . . common sense," Creagh wrote in her report. "Yet it is also clear that this danger was not perceived by the health-care professionals; their collective experience told them that the danger was the loss of the IV site."

Creagh's report included 21 suggestions for improving the safety of patients under the age of four. These include attaching tubes or wires only when required for immediate medical purposes and increasing observation of youngsters hooked up to tubes or wires by assigning one staff member to every two of these patients. Also, patients should be placed in glass-walled rooms close to nurses.

The judge also recommended the recording of all tangles on medical charts and reporting incidents that lead to injuries to major databases, so other institutes can learn from them. In February 2001, Sharon wrote to the editor of the Edmonton Journal, "It is our belief that incidents involving IV tubing and infants occur much more frequently than commonly thought; however, these incidents are not formalized in a report or a patient's chart."

Creagh commended Capital Health for establishing new policies to deal with tubes and tangling before the release of her report. She did, however, criticize the health authority for the lack of information Carter's parents received after he died. "Prompt and empathetic communication is required," the judge wrote.

Sharon said, "Overall, hospital officials were reluctant to discuss anything with us. For several days, they even refused to give me a copy of Carter's hospital charts. I had to go to the hospital and sit in the nursing manager's office before I was given a copy. And then, there were differences in what was recorded to have happened during the last hour at the Royal Alexandra Hospital between this copy and the copy submitted by the hospital to the Public Fatality Inquiry."

In November 2000, the Tapps filed a $4.2 million lawsuit. They thought the threat of monetary loss and unfavourable publicity would cause the hospital to improve infant IV care. The lawsuit was eventually settled out of court following the close of the fatality inquiry.

During the preparation of this story, Dr. Daniel Garros, a pediatric intensive care physician, who briefly saw Carter in the ICU, provided insights into the interaction between the hospital and the Tapp family.

> Every health-care professional directly or indirectly involved with this unfortunate and extremely sad circumstance was very distraught, to say the least. I even witnessed a key person in the hospital administration coming to tears because that person wanted to go straight to the family at their home right after the fact and say that we were all so sorry for what had happened. Unfortunately, the *modus operandi* at that time dictated, perhaps even based on a lawyer's advice, that nobody from the hospital side should do that. It was so sad and in fact revolting to hear that someone was prevented from doing the right thing! Fortunately that culture has changed already, but nobody at the time had the knowledge that it was a risk until it happened the first time. Hence, we decided with utmost respect to Carter's family to write a report for a peer-reviewed medical journal.

The report was a paper Garros and three colleagues, two physicians and a nurse, published in the June 2003 issue of the journal *Pediatrics* on the circumstances of Carter's death and of the non-fatal strangulation involving IV tubing of an eight-and-a-half-month-old boy.[2] It is the first report in the medical literature of strangulation with intravenous tubing in children. The authors provided recommendations on active prevention strategy and included a photograph of Reilly's IV stabilizer. The article had an immediate impact. Pediatric centres throughout Canada and the United States and elsewhere contacted Garros asking for more information on protocol and the stabilizer. Even today, years after publication, he continues to receive requests for information.

The Tapps Speak

The Tapps offer their sincere thanks to the continuing support of their family and friends, to Eleanor Olszewski for the exemplary way in which she presented their concerns at the Public Fatality Inquiry and to members of the media who allowed them to tell their tragic story in their own time and at their own pace. They also recognize the many people who have worked to prevent this tragedy from happening to other families.

To parents everywhere they say, "Please hug your children for us and keep them close."

The Whisper

Theresa Malloy-Miller

Dan Miller, an active, apparently healthy 17-year-old died suddenly in the early hours of January 9, 2003, 12 hours after being admitted to an Ontario teaching hospital. The autopsy report said the immediate cause of death was an enlarged heart, resulting from a subacute ongoing non-specific inflammation of the heart muscles. But what role did the administration of two powerful drugs three minutes before Dan stopped breathing play in his death? Or the failure to recheck Dan's electrolyte balance after being seen for enteritis and dehydration in the emergency room three days before his death? Or the nurses not acknowledging the importance of Dan's falling blood pressure and blaming the low readings on the equipment? Only because Dan's parents, Tim Miller and Theresa Malloy-Miller, insisted on finding answers to these and other questions were the circumstances of their son's death investigated, errors revealed and at least some steps taken to prevent recurrence. Eventually, Tim and Theresa realized their only hope of letting go of their anger and seeking a way to forgive was to work toward positive change. Dan's voice is the constant whisper that has compelled them to become leaders in the patient safety movement. This is Dan's story as told by his mother.

A grade 12 student strong in math and science, Dan was well on his way to realizing his dream of studying biochemistry at the University of Waterloo. Not long before he became ill, he had sent in his application and was looking forward to being at university with his older brother and best friend, Ben. Dan was well liked for his kindness and easygoing manner, and he enjoyed hanging out with his friends. He played electric guitar, was teaching himself to play the drums and had a considerable aptitude for drawing. At various times, he played lacrosse, hockey and soccer. In all ways, Dan was a healthy, active teenager.

January 4 – January 9, 2003

On Saturday, January 4, 2003, Dan started to feel unwell and by Sunday evening he was vomiting every 45 minutes. On Monday, January 6, we called TeleHealth Ontario and were advised to take Dan to the emergency room at a local hospital. He was much sicker than Tim or I had ever seen him. The ER wasn't busy when Dan and I arrived, and he was seen quickly by nursing staff and then a doctor. The nurse recorded Dan's heart rate as 140 beats per minute. The doctor remarked that he couldn't believe that it was that rapid and checked it himself. He diagnosed Dan as having enteritis and being dehydrated. The doctor said Dan would be started on fluid replacement intravenously and once he had voided he could go home. Over the next four and a half hours, Dan received 3.6 litres of normal saline.

When he was admitted, Dan's blood was drawn and the electrolyte levels were tested. No other blood work was done that day. Only later did we learn that the levels of three of the electrolyte tests were abnormal — the potassium was abnormally high, as was the anion gap level, and the level of bicarbonate was lower than normal. There was no reassessment of electrolyte levels after Dan had received the large quantity of saline. Eventually, Dan voided a small amount of urine, 100 ml, and was released from the ER with instructions to drink Gatorade. He was sent home with green hospital basins, because he was still vomiting.

Dan did not improve during the evening of the day of his release or on the next day. On Tuesday, he not only continued to vomit, but his breathing became unusual. After failing to get an appointment with our family doctor and calling TeleHealth Ontario for the second time, I took Dan to the ER on the afternoon of Wednesday, January 8.

Upon our arrival at the ER, the triage nurse said that Dan "just might have to wait it out." The nurse also said, in a very offhand manner, that the doctor would see Dan, since he was already there. After these remarks, I felt foolish for bringing him back. This pattern of not recognizing the seriousness of Dan's condition continued.

Dan was seen by four more doctors as he progressed from the ER to the children's in-patient floor and finally to the pediatric critical care unit (PCCU). His father and I kept asking about his rapid heart rate, in the range of 132 bpm, and his odd breathing. To our knowledge, these were never considered indicative of cardiac problems, but only as symptoms associated with dehydration. A heart murmur was noted on his chart as a new finding, but we were not told of this at the time.

Dan's blood pressure was continuing to fall. This was attributed to vagaries of the equipment and never considered to be a serious sign until shortly before Dan died. The doctors decided that Dan had hepatitis. He was given another 1.5 litres of saline. A medical student asked Dan if he had gained weight. Dan answered, "What do you think? I have been throwing up for four days." The student did not tell Dan that his chart indicated a weight gain of 3.5 pounds between his first and second visit to the ER.

Eventually, Dan was admitted to the seventh floor of the children's ward. His blood pressure continued to be low, at one point being recorded as 58/35. Tim and I asked if that was normal, to which question the nurse replied, "It is normal for that machine." This was the second time that the nurses failed to recognize the importance of faulty equipment and inaccurate readings. The nurses kept changing machines and never told us just how serious the readings were.

Dan wanted to sleep and said he wouldn't be able to "if we kept staring at him." We left him around 11:30 p.m. in order to get some sleep ourselves. The nurses reassured us that Dan was fine and there were lots of doctors around. Shortly afterward, he was given another litre of normal saline intravenously.

At 2:15 a.m. on Thursday, January 9, we received a call informing us that Dan had been transferred to the critical care unit. The nurse said on the phone that Dan was still okay and they had better equipment in the critical care unit. I grabbed a change of clothes for Dan and we left immediately for the hospital.

According to his hospital file, Dan was transferred to the critical care unit around 2:00 a.m., because of laboured breathing and worsening acidosis. When Dan arrived in the care unit, his blood pressure was too low to register on the blood pressure machine. However, he was still allowed to transfer himself into bed. He was alert and talking about going to university.

At 2:25 a.m., he was given sedation (fentanyl and midazolam) as ordered by a resident. This was done despite a nurse asking twice if there was any concern about administering these medications, considering that Dan's blood pressure could not be attained. The resident dismissed these remarks as a query from a junior nurse and insisted the medications be given. Dan stopped breathing three minutes after the nurse intravenously injected the drugs. We arrived as the doctors were trying to revive him. Dan was pronounced dead at 3:50 a.m.

Upon investigation, I found that three minutes falls within the time frame given for the action of these medications when administered intravenously. According to the hospital's own drug guidelines posted on its website at that time, the adverse effects of midazolam include respiratory depression, especially when combined with narcotics. Fentynal is a narcotic and its adverse effects include slowing the beating rate of the heart. Both drugs lower blood pressure.

It was never explained to us either at the time or in subsequent investigations and meetings with doctors and hospital officials why Dan required sedation at all, let alone with such potentially dangerous drugs.

The Next Four Years — Reviews, Complaints, Appeals, Frustration, Disappointment and a Beacon of Hope

The suddenness of Dan's death and its enormity left our family reeling. After several weeks, we asked to meet with doctors from the hospital.

A meeting was arranged for February 19, 2003. Little did we realize at the time that by taking this first step to find answers about why Dan died we had started on an arduous journey that would last for the next several years. At the end, we would have only partial answers and be frustrated and disappointed. Our perseverance, however, did lead to some changes for the better.

At the hospital meeting, the doctors told us there was nothing that could have been done for Dan. I remember the physicians saying that Dan had the "worst case possible of myocarditis," and he would have died no matter what they did. During this meeting, my sister, who had been an ER nurse for several years, reviewed his file and noticed that he had been given midazolam and fentanyl. When asked why these drugs had been used, the doctors appeared to be uncomfortable and said that it is routine in pediatrics to use these drugs for sedation. In time, we would come to understand the significance of my sister's question.

We had many concerns after that meeting and arranged to get a copy of Dan's medical file. Our concerns increased after reviewing the file, and we spoke with and then wrote to the local coroner involved with Dan's case. The coroner asked the hospital to investigate further. We provided an extensive list of questions to the relevant hospital administrators. Our request to be included in the review was denied.

The results of the hospital review were sent to us in early June 2003; it said that the care provided to Dan met a reasonable standard. Shortly thereafter, we met with medical and administrative staff to discuss the review. We had many questions, most of which were not answered. However, we did receive an answer by omission to one critically important question. When we asked if all present had reviewed Dan's medical file, no one answered.

There were four points in the review that particularly concerned us. First, the only reference to sedation drugs in the review was "use of sedation and analgesia are so common as to not be worthy of comment." Fentanyl and midazolam were not mentioned in the Death Summary prepared by the attending physician, which formed part of Dan's medical file. We learned this omission was because the attending physician relied on the resident's notes of January 9, in which he did not mention ordering the drugs. The nurse's charted notes, however, are quite explicit about the drugs. She wrote: "F & M given as ordered by Dr.____ by myself. Asked Dr.___ x 2 if there was any concern administering these drugs if Daniel's BP not attainable. Stated he wanted them given. Approximately 3 min p administration of midazolam Daniel became apneic."

Second, there was a discrepancy concerning the severity of myocarditis. At the meeting in February, we were told that Dan had severe myocarditis, yet the autopsy report contained this statement: "The intensity of the inflammation is relatively mild but sufficient to define ongoing myocarditis." According to the autopsy report, the immediate cause of death was dilated cardiomyopathy due to subacute ongoing non-specific myocarditis.

Third, we discovered a disturbing error in the Death Summary; it listed *illicit drug and toxin ingestion* as high on the list for probable cause of death. We were dumbfounded when we read this. Dan had not had an opportunity to ingest alcohol and even if he had, he would have vomited it before it could have entered his bloodstream. We pursued this matter with the local coroner and requested that Dan's final blood sample be tested. It came back negative for alcohol. We then demanded that the Death Summary be corrected. An addendum was written to correct the error.

And fourth, it is stated in the Death Summary that Dan was felt to be doing better when he left the ER on January 6. There is no recorded comment in his hospital chart that supports this statement.

The local coroner agreed with the hospital review and felt his involvement in the case was completed. We questioned whether this coroner was able to discharge his duty of speaking for the dead in an unbiased manner, because of apparent conflicts of interest which were never declared to us. First, the coroner's family practice was associated with the hospital, and he wrote to us using hospital letterhead, not that of the Ontario coroners service. We discovered on the internet that at this time he also sat on the council of the Canadian Medical Protection Association, which provides its physician members with medical-legal advice, risk management education and legal assistance related to their clinical practice. Specifically, the local coroner chaired the committee that determines the amount of legal assistance doctors will receive. The regional coroner to whom the local coroner reported told us that it is not unusual for doctors who are also coroners to be involved in these types of activities.

Near the end of June 2003, we submitted a request for a review of Dan's case to the Pediatric Review Committee of the Office of the Chief Coroner of Ontario. John Lewis, whose daughter Claire died as a result of an adverse event in Hamilton on October 2001, helped us prepare the request. We also registered complaints with the College of Physicians and Surgeons of Ontario (CPSO) and the College of Nurses of Ontario (CNO).

The report of the pediatric death review committee, which was issued in October 2003, verified many of our concerns. It said that, given the results of the blood tests, the diagnosis of enteritis and dehydration on January 6 was questionable. All the doctors who reviewed information provided by the committee stated that they would not have discharged Dan on January 6 without further investigation. The report also said that the diagnosis of hepatitis made on January 8 was not consistent with laboratory results and that Dan was given a significant amount of IV fluid on the same day without any clear rationale for its use. Furthermore, the report stated that the finding of "unexplained acidosis seems to have been under-appreciated and there seems to have been inadequate input into the possible diagnosis and treatment at the staff physician level at the time of admission to the pediatric ward." In other words, there was not adequate supervision of the resident doctor.

The review found the administration of the sedation medicine to be inappropriate. The committee members were concerned that hospital officials had written in the letter of June 10 to us that "use of sedation and analgesia are so common as to not be worthy of comment." They were also concerned that questions related to medication use were not included in the Death Summary. As well, they found that the resident doctor had not followed hospital medication guidelines.

The report emphasized that the foregoing issues were not addressed in the review done by the hospital and discussed with us in June.

The pediatric review committee recommended that abnormal laboratory tests be repeated before the patient is discharged, that medication guidelines that are already in place should be followed and that the hospital examine its internal death review process. The committee invited a representative of the hospital to become a member.

Early in September 2003, we were informed that another meeting with hospital administrators was being planned. In late November, the Canadian Medical Protective Association advised the doctors associated with Daniel's case not to meet with us any further. At this point, hospital administrators felt there was no reason for us to meet again, because doctors are private practitioners and the hospital was not able to "comment or adjudicate on medical decisions made by pediatricians or internists." Our lengthy list of questions remained unanswered. From all indications, the hospital medical staff continued to consider that the care they had given Dan was reasonable.

Tim and I were distraught, as we felt that this tragedy could happen again — a frightening and frustrating possibility. We remained confused about who had the authority to effect needed and specific changes in health-care practice. All we wanted was a clear and truthful acknowledgement of how our son died in a facility that portrayed itself as "leading edge." We wanted to know what changes would be made and if these changes would be enduring.

For several years, we wrote letters to politicians, radio stations and newspapers. We also corresponded extensively with the College of Physicians and Surgeons of Ontario and the Ontario College of Nurses concerning the complaints we had made against six doctors and seven nurses in June 2003. We did not lay a complaint against the nurse who injected Dan with the fentynal and midazolam, because without her charted notes, we would never have known the possibility that those drugs played a role in Dan's death.

The complaint process with the colleges was a gruelling experience. This is a brief summary of our dealings with the CPSO.

- July 2003: Complaint laid; repeated responses by doctors and ourselves.
- August 2004: CPSO report issued; we appealed to Health Professions Appeal and Review Board.
- May 2005: HPARB report issued and sent to CPSO.
- August 2005: One physician appealed, which stopped second review by CPSO.
- June 2006: CPSO issued report on second review, which occurred only because of our persistent efforts.

In a letter dated July 14, 2006, the college generally upheld the decisions made by the appeal and review board. Details were added to the written cautions given to two physicians. The caution to one doctor was reworded to make it a more understandable and accurate statement. The college did not take action against a fourth physician and stated, "Regrettably, the initial presentation of Daniel's illness was not easily diagnosed, and this was compounded by certain inadvertent errors which together contributed to the tragic outcome."

The complaint process with the College of Nurses involved submission of documents, interviews of nurses and reviews. An initial report was issued in July 2004. The report said two nurses had received written cautions, two were to appear before the complaints committee and two were referred to the quality assurance committee for review. In November 2004, we received a report from the CNO summarizing the process and the information collected, but not the exact wording of the cautions. We weren't pleased with the report, but did not appeal. We were simply too exhausted.

The review processes by the two colleges were excruciatingly painful for us and at the end we did not have a sense of satisfaction. Neither one addressed needed system changes, because they are so individually focused. Both the CPSO processes and CNO processes are very time-limited and apparently lack the ability to explore the actions and procedures that led to the adverse events in Dan's care. Tim and I walked away from both processes with a tired, empty feeling. We did gain more information about what had happened; unfortunately, we remain uncertain that these reviews ever led to meaningful change.

A positive outcome was that the college reviews provided a means to communicate with the health professionals involved. At the appeals and review board meeting for the physicians, one doctor spoke of the courses he had taken and how he had changed his practice after Dan's death. He said that he thinks about Daniel every day and can't imagine when he will no longer do so. At the end of his presentation, we shook hands with him and wished him well. He wept with relief. This has remained a treasured interaction and a beacon of light for us.

Working for Change and a Change of Heart at the Hospital

Tim and I realized that we needed to let go of our anger and seek a way to forgive. Our only hope of achieving this was to work toward positive change. Dan would have expected no less of us.

One of my first steps was to attend conferences and workshops on patient safety. In March 2006, I participated in a focus group for the Ontario Patient Safety Task Force. I also went to an Ontario Hospital Association Conference on patient safety. I was desperately trying to understand how to assure safe medical care. At those meetings and since, I talk to whomever I can about the need for a consumer health group.

In the summer of 2006, I received an email about a patient safety conference to be held in Vancouver. Of particular interest to me was a patient discussion group. I contacted Ryan Sidorchuk, leader of the group, who invited me to come to Vancouver. At the conference, I was selected to be among 22 Canadian Patients for Patient Safety Champions. These champions were the initial members of what became Patients for Patient Safety Canada, which is part of a global network under the auspices of the World Alliance for Patient Safety, an initiative of the World Health Organization. Patients for Patient Safety Canada is now a working group of the Canadian Patient Safety

Institute. The institute was created in December 2003 by Health Canada, which provides funding.

After the conference in Vancouver, I contacted our local paper, which ran a story primarily about Dan and not about the patient safety group, as I had hoped. I, along with the director of quality and patient safety at the hospital where Dan died, subsequently participated in a radio interview in November 2006. The topic was the need for dis-closure of adverse events. We were quite surprised by the director's concluding statement, "As always, the hospital continues to want to speak to this family if that is what they desire."

A few weeks later, we received an email from the new hospital CEO asking to meet with us. A meeting was arranged with the CEO and other hospital administrators in February 2007. At that time we received a verbal apology and the first genuine disclosure of the circumstances associated with Dan's case. We were also told of the changes that the hospital had made. These changes included:

- Establishing a required set of parameters and blood tests that must be retested prior to discharge of children from the ER.
- Giving authority to all staff members to ensure these tests are repeated.
- Establishing a standard protocol for children who require fluid resuscitation.
- Increasing education for both medical and nursing staff about myocarditis.
- Adding four charge-nurse positions in the ER to support nurses so they can more confidently advocate for families.
- Updating and standardizing thermometers and blood pressure machines.
- Reviewing and clarifying pediatric critical care unit admission procedures and guidelines for administration of analgesics and sedatives, and including them in resident education in a more formal manner.
- Appointing a representative of the hospital to the Pediatric Death Review Committee.

Other changes at the hospital included:

- Adding rapid response teams which can be activated by any member of the care team or family members.
- Focusing on respect among team members.
- Improving communication between members of the care team to ensure accurate and complete transfer of patient information.
- Emphasizing patient safety.
- Developing a disclosure policy.

In October 2007, Tim and I presented Dan's story at the first Patient Safety Conference held in London, Ontario. I am now a member of the planning committee. Tim and I told Dan's story during Patient Safety Week in October 2008 and at the Healthcare Insurance Reciprocal of Canada conference in November 2009. The insurance reciprocal is the largest health-care liability insurer in Canada.

Seven years after Dan's death, Tim and I continue to look for ways to make health care safer for all. We believe that safer care will come with true family-centred care. This will require accountability, insightful leadership, respectful communication between all members of the health-care team and families, and the use of best practices.

Vance's Gift

Donna Davis

On a cold March morning in 2002, 19-year-old Vance Davis rolled his Ford *Expedition* on a highway in southeast Saskatchewan. Five days later, he died in hospital from traumatic brain injuries sustained in the accident. The suffering of Vance's parents, Jack and Donna Davis, was made worse by knowing that more could have been done to save their son's life and compounded by the health region's refusal to accept any responsibility. Poor communication with nursing staff was a major concern of the Davis family. Donna, a licensed practical nurse, former ambulance attendant and first responder facilitator, repeatedly brought signs of Vance's deteriorating condition to the attention of those overseeing his care. Among the coroner's recommendations was that nurses must listen to family members and communicate their concerns to physicians in a timely manner. As time passed, Jack and Donna resumed their lives, but they couldn't "just move on" as well-meaning associates encouraged them to do. They wanted an apology, an acknowledgement of responsibility and a way to help ensure that these circumstances would not be repeated. Five and a half years after Vance's death, events began to unfold that would lead to the fulfillment of their wishes. Here Donna tells of some of those events and her extensive involvement in patient safety in Canada and elsewhere.

Times Change

In 2007, I learned that the Sun Country Health Region in Saskatchewan, where I have been employed for my entire nursing career, was going to hold its first-ever patient safety conference. The organizers wanted a patient story about an experience of things going wrong. They sent staff a memorandum asking if we knew of anyone who might have such a story. I knew Vance's story could help health-care providers learn better ways to care for patients and their families, so I spoke with members of the organizing committee. Although we worked in the same health region, they had no idea of what had happened to Vance. I presented our son's story for the first time at the Patient Safety Conference held October 7, 2007, in Weyburn, Saskatchewan. This marked the start of a journey that has taken me to more conferences than I can count and allowed me to reach a multitude of caring health-care providers who want to give excellent care. It has also given me the opportunity to speak to medical and nursing students at an impressionable stage in their lives. Along the way, I have met many patients and families who have experienced adverse events and are working to make our health-care system safer for everyone.

Volunteering to participate in that first conference quickly led to something Jack and I had wanted so badly, which was recognition from authorities that Vance had not received adequate treatment. It also led to a supportive friendship with a woman whose words helped us to heal. As plans were being finalized for the conference, an organizer mentioned to another presenter, Paula Beard, that I would be on the agenda. Paula, an operations manager with the Canadian Patient Safety Institute, had been the risk manager who conducted the case review of Vance's care. The review's eventual report, which gave no indication of any breakdown in Vance's care, devastated Jack and me. I wrote letters to many people, from the chief officer of nursing at the hospital to the Minister of Health, telling them of our disappointment in the results of the review. In response, we received a letter from the health authority's client care coordinator informing us that any further communication would be through the hospital's lawyers.

Paula asked the organizer if I was Vance Davis's mother. Upon being told I was, she called immediately. Her first words were "Donna, we failed Vance in our care of him and we failed you as a family." It was as if a huge weight had been lifted off my shoulders. Finally! I had validation of what I had known to be true all along. We talked for two hours, sharing what had happened during those tragic four days. I could not wait to tell Jack and my daughters what Paula had said. They, too, rejoiced.

Paula and I met for the first time at the conference. The friendship that developed is an example of how people can move beyond divisive circumstances and work together for a common goal of benefiting others. I needed the validation she provided in order to go forward after the conference and tell Vance's story to a wider audience. At the conclusion of that first conference, a woman said, "Donna, it must be so hard to tell Vance's story."

I replied, "It was harder not to."

In 2007, Patients for Patient Safety Canada (PFPSC), a patient-led program of the CPSI, was in its fledgling stages. The group was being developed under the umbrella of the World Health Organization, which recognized the patient voice as an untapped resource and was encouraging the development of patient-led organizations worldwide. Paula suggested that I might like to become involved. I agreed immediately. I knew as a nurse working in the system and as a mother who had experienced harm in the system that I had to be part of influencing change by telling Vance's story. This organization could provide the venue to do that and, I hoped, much more. I was soon accepted as a member.

Patients for Patient Safety Canada initially had only a handful of members, but grew by word of mouth and with the help of a little marketing. In November 2007, 20 new champions of patient safety were designated at an in-country workshop spearheaded by WHO and held in Winnipeg. Like me, they were people who had experienced harm to themselves or to their loved ones, often with fatal outcomes. These people wanted to direct their grief, anger and sense of injustice in a way that would result in safer care for every patient. Patients for

Patient Safety Canada provided them with a way to create change by partnering with health organizations and providers as co-producers of strategies to improve patient care.

I was elected to the first board of directors and then as one of the organization's first co-chairs. Katarina Busija of Toronto was the other co-chair. I was humbled and honoured to come from a tiny little hamlet in Saskatchewan and be chosen as a leader of this group. This was my chance to see that Vance and all the others who had died or been harmed had a voice, and to try to ensure the lessons learned from their experiences were carried forward.

The Power of Stories

But first, with Paula's backing, I had some personal issues to resolve. I had to try to renew my relationship with the Regina Qu'Appelle Health Region (RQHR) in order to achieve a mutual understanding regarding Vance's death. The climate of health care had changed in the years since Vance's death with the inception of the Canadian Patient Safety Institute, the release of the Baker/Norton study that brought to light the number of deaths and harmful events in the Canadian health-care system and the release of the Canadian Disclosure Guidelines by CPSI. Without Paula's influence and my affiliation with PFPSC and WHO, I don't think I would have been viewed as anything other than an angry mother who wanted someone to blame. Little did the members of the health region know that my anger had long ago been replaced by a sadness, hurt and the sense that I had been betrayed by my peers. I had also long suspected that nothing was going to change. A meeting with the health region could provide a chance to restore my faith in my peers and in the system itself. Eventually a meeting was agreed upon. I was scared and apprehensive, just as I thought they might be.

The meeting, which was held on March 31, 2008, one day before the sixth anniversary of Vance's death, was the first time the RQHR had met with a family to discuss an adverse event. Disclosure was a scary, unknown entity to everyone. The region felt they had to set boundaries, and in doing so caused more harm to me and my family. We received an email from the risk manager giving us a list of what they would and would not do at the meeting. It was a long list which included statements such as we will not apologize, we will not accept any responsibility for Vance's death, we will not have the frontline workers there, we will not have the physicians there, and we will not share the case review. Also, we were given only one hour in which to present our case.

I phoned Paula and she told me to take what was offered. She assured me that when we started telling Vance's story those present would give us the time we needed. How true this proved to be. At the beginning of the meeting, we sensed defensiveness, skepticism and hostility. We had to remind the risk manager to let us tell our story. The mood in the room changed almost immediately when I showed a video of Vance and started speaking about what we had seen and experienced at his bedside. At the end of the meeting, one of the people present said this was the most disturbing story he had ever heard. We received the apologies and expressions of remorse we had so badly needed six years before. While we appreciated all of them, they fell short, because none came from the people who cared for Vance in the last days of his life.

As a direct result of that meeting, three health-care providers vowed that they would make improvements in their departments, so that they would never again hear of a tragedy like Vance's. They modified an electronic patient reporting system in the emergency room. Concerns regarding a patient's condition would prompt a red, flashing stop sign called "Vance's Stop Sign." This lets caregivers know there is something that demands their attention before the patient is discharged or transferred. Anyone — porter, nurse, family member — can activate the sign. When I visited the ER recently, I saw six stop signs on the board. Vance's story is also being used in the hospital as a learning tool during employee orientation.

In 2008, I began approaching health-care educational institutions in Saskatchewan about the possibility of telling Vance's story. The University of Saskatchewan medical school was the first to accept my offer. Although pleased, I was also nervous about my ability to tell the story and wondered how it would be received. On a stormy winter day, I made the six-hour drive to Saskatoon. I talked to Vance most of the way, drawing strength from knowing he would be proud of what I was doing. Once I was standing before the students and started to speak, my nervousness vanished and the story just flowed. Afterward, many students spoke with me. "I will never forget this story and the lessons you have shared from it. I will carry this with me throughout my career," one student said. "Every medical student needs to hear this story," said another. I was proud that in death Vance was still able to help others.

The university recognized the value of patient and family voices in educating students about the reality of medical harm and has invited me back every year since. As with most of the other presentations I give, I receive a modest reimbursement for expenses and volunteer my time. I can't think of a better way to spend my time than reaching young health-care professionals at the beginning of their careers.

On average, I give at least a dozen presentations a year to a wide spectrum of groups and organizations, including pharmacists, nurses, regional health authorities and ministries of health. Most of these presentations are in person, but some are done through webinars. In this way, I can reach people across the country who log on at their convenience. I believe my association with the World Health Organization as a Patient Safety Champion and the backing of the Canadian Patient Safety Institute has helped me to become an effective spokesperson.

Committees and Working Groups

As a member and co-chair of Patients for Patient Safety Canada, I have served on various committees and working groups, including the groups to develop the PFPSC Disclosure Principles and a brochure for the public regarding the newly implemented Safe Surgical Checklist. I also sit on the Membership Committee.

Currently, I am involved as the patient representative on the CPSI Teamwork and Communication Working group. As the coroner indicated in his report, a breakdown in communication played a key role in the circumstances associated with Vance's death. After his death, a provincial alert about the importance of clear communication regarding the exchange of information during handoffs between shifts was sent to all health regions. I was pleased to be asked to serve on this working group. The teamwork and communication group was also instrumental in revising the Canadian Disclosure Guidelines.

My goals for the regional, provincial, national and international health-care conferences I attend are to not only share my experiences, but also to learn from some of the foremost leaders in patient safety. Paula Beard, Hugh McLeod, Michael Gardam, Dan Florizone, Rob Robson and all my fellow PFPSC members are just a few of the Canadian patient safety champions I hold in high esteem. Don Berwick, Aaron Lazar and Jim Conway are some of my heroes in the United States. From these people and an increasing number of others, I derive the knowledge and enthusiasm to continue my journey.

I have petitioned various groups to include the patient/family voice in all aspects of health-care improvements and policy. My argument is, "Who better to ask what is needed than the people who are at the receiving end of the care?" I am pleased to say that patients and their families are now included on several Saskatchewan Ministry of Health committees. In addition, while at round-table discussions with health-care executives and managers, I see first-hand a genuine desire to hear the patient/family perspective.

After Vance died, a doctor I work with told me, "Donna, you can let this make you bitter or you can let it make you better." Although my family and I were bitter and angry after this tragedy, we eventually realized what Dr. Botha said was true.

Vance's gift to me was the ability to make things better for other people and to honour him while doing so. Vance was known as a "fixer" in his young life and he remains a "fixer" in death. His story reaches the hearts and minds of many people and drives change. In addition, we cannot forget the people who are alive today because Vance's organs "fixed" them. Through these gifts of life, this strong, hard-working young man lives on.

Claire's Story

Raeline McGrath

Following the death of their nine-year-old daughter in a pediatric intensive care unit, Raeline McGrath and her husband, David Smith, had questions concerning Claire's care. The situation was complicated by Raeline's employment as a registered nurse in the same program. If they sought answers to their questions, Raeline knew without a doubt she would be labelled as ungrateful and seen as a mother trying to blame someone for her daughter's death. Their commitment to Claire, however, was greater than their concern about these consequences. Raeline and David approached the health authority, Eastern Regional Health Authority of Newfoundland and Labrador, which ordered an external review. The review finding of a preventable death increased tensions between her former colleagues and Raeline, who now works as a resident care manager in a long-term care facility. Eastern Health apologized to David and Raeline and worked with Raeline to develop a presentation, "Claire's Story," which is being used widely as a teaching tool, regionally, provincially and nationally. Raeline also wrote an article of the same name which was published in Canadian Nurse. That article forms the first part of this story. In the second part, Raeline provides additional insights into the circumstances of Claire's death, her feelings as a mother and a nurse, and the fundamental importance of honest and open communication between families and health-care providers when things go wrong. Because Claire had such a remarkable mother who was fortunate

163

to work in a co-operative health authority, she leaves a legacy of hope and understanding for both families and organizations.

Claire's Story, *Canadian Nurse*, October 2009[1]

It was mid-afternoon on postoperative day 13, and "quiet hour" in the pediatric intensive care unit. Things were unchanged, still *critically unstable . . . only one system involved.* Parents are not usually permitted in the PICU at this time of day, but I was sitting by my daughter's bed. No one had come to remove me. Maybe they felt bad for us; we had already spent many hours away from her that day during rounds and while a chest tube was being inserted.

I had an "aha" moment: *Claire may actually die in here, she may never open her eyes again.* But I immediately switched to the familiar, practical and prepared mode that had sustained me for the past nine and half years: *Well, if Claire is going to die, I'd better tell her about heaven, just in case, just on the off chance such a place exists.* After all, my family and I had long guided Claire through events and expectations by using simple explanations.

The oscillator beat loudly next to me, and the beeps from the many drips that were keeping her alive were steady. I removed the earphone that was playing her favourite music. Two nurses looked on as I squeezed in between the oscillator, the bed and the chest tube. I put my mouth up close to my little girl's ear. I am grateful to those nurses who allowed me to stay with Claire that afternoon and explain what heaven was . . . just in case. Three days later, we consented to withdraw the ventilator that kept Claire alive, and she died.

The Road Less Travelled

Claire was diagnosed with trisomy 13, or Patau syndrome, in the months following her birth. It is a life-shortening syndrome. We discovered through an international support organization that not all children with trisomy 13 die young and that the presentation for each child is unique. The future was uncertain, but we were "good to go" with what lay ahead.

At the age of nine, Claire was considered a long-term survivor. She had severe global developmental delay and was completely non-verbal, but she understood most of what was said to her as long as the concepts were basic and familiar. When she was in the mood, she used pictures to communicate. She required constant supervision and 24-hour care, but she was medically healthy. She rarely missed a day of school. Our goal was to keep her safe and happy, and we took great care in doing just that. We vowed to see Claire's life through with her. We often wondered how her end would finally come, but never thought it would play out as it did in the PICU.

Navigating the PICU

In fall 2006, Claire's doctor noted a scoliosis of 13 degrees on an x-ray. At home, Claire seemed to want to walk less and less and began to have trouble swallowing. The next fall, an MRI of her head and spine was done. The scoliosis had progressed to 46 degrees. A Chiari I malformation was diagnosed. Her spine was disintegrating. The Chiari I had to be surgically corrected or paralysis would spread.

Our PICU journey began. Claire had multiple behaviour problems and we, like her trusted neurosurgeon, felt that her habit of head-banging when agitated would seriously hinder her recovery in the immediate post-op period. The intensivist and anesthesiologist were consulted. It was in Claire's best interest, it was decided, that she remain sedated, intubated and ventilated in the PICU for at least seven days. After a successful neurosurgical procedure, and several wonderful hours of apparently good health, judging by sensor readings and appearance, Claire developed pneumonia and, according to one intensivist, acute respiratory distress syndrome (ARDS).

During those 16 days in the PICU, our emotions took a wild ride with stops at relief, disbelief, uncertainty and heartbreak as Claire's condition worsened, got better and worsened in cycles. Within the first 48 hours, the No Code conversations began. Again and again, quietly and loudly, publicly and privately, over and over, I confirmed to the medical staff that yes, Claire was a *Full Code*. Of course, she was a Full Code! We were incredulous that anything else was being considered. Our wishes were obvious and simple: *We want Claire's treatment plan exhausted. We need to be kept informed every step of the way, and we will decide together if it is time to stop.*

It was accepted practice in the PICU to move parents from the bedside to the other side of the locked door during multi-disciplinary rounds, shift changes and invasive procedures. We were often denied entrance to the PICU when Claire's condition suddenly worsened. We would sit on the floor and wait for permission to enter once the team inside the unit had a handle on what was happening. We were always allowed back into the unit, but we did not feel that we were ever fully invited into the difficult and complex conversation about her care that took place in offices, behind closed doors and at her bedside when we weren't there.

Claire needed all that the PICU had to offer, but she also needed us to be her voice. We had expected to be partners in Claire's care. We understood that decisions in critical care environments are often based on probabilities rather than certainties, and we would have put stock in the physicians' thoughts and opinions. But they were selective in what they shared with us. Maybe they were afraid that we would not understand. Maybe they worried that acknowledging the uncertainties would undermine our confidence in their abilities. That would not have been the case.

Revelations and Reactions

One of the intensivists who cared for our daughter felt that Claire's tragic and unexpected course through the PICU was somehow related to trisomy 13. I suppose there is some truth to this; we wonder if those who worked so hard to keep Claire alive derailed those efforts by falling into the trap of labelling her. Claire acquired a number of dangerous labels in the PICU: acute respiratory distress syndrome, trisomy 13, No Code, do not resuscitate. And *futile* may have been another of the words on that list. Tragic decisions about Claire's care were made because of these labels. But assigning them might have been easier than grappling with uncertainty about what to do or say next.

At the time, we believed that we had an excellent, transparent relationship with the PICU staff. After Claire died, we sent thank-you cards to them, and we publicly acknowledged their efforts. We hung a picture of Claire on the memory wall in the PICU to mark her time there. The caption read, "Well cared for in the PICU for 16 days." This was how we very much wanted, and needed, Claire's story to end.

But we had questions. There were events that did not sit right with us. Two of the intensivists were patient with us and answered our questions as best they could. But ultimately, we still had concerns. The health region brought in a team of out-of-province reviewers to examine Claire's time in the PICU. The revelations were shocking. We learned that Claire had not been cared for in the manner that we expected or that she deserved. The PICU staff members were hurt and angry that we could not accept that everything medically possible had been done — what more could we have wanted? Why were we seemingly so *ungrateful*? Being a nurse, shouldn't I have understood the limits of medical intervention? I too was hurt and angry. Why couldn't the PICU team see me as a mother driven to understand why her daughter died so unexpectedly on their watch? Why couldn't they understand that I was a mother first and a nurse second? Didn't they want to understand the mistakes that had been made and to learn from them? Claire's journey and death in the PICU metastasized into a mass of indignation and denial. A nurse removed Claire's picture from the memory wall. Already devastated by our daughter's death, we now had to cope with the review findings and the reactions of the staff we had trusted so completely.

We received three formal apologies — all from nurses — for mistakes and deficiencies in our daughter's care. The first came from the director of the program, on behalf of the health region. Her sadness and regret were sincere, and we accepted her apology. The second came from someone who had spent many an hour at Claire's bedside, working hard to keep her alive. Her tears flowed freely as she expressed her regret for any involvement she might have unknowingly had in our daughter's death. As I listened, I thought of this nurse's courage. Would I have been able to apologize in this way if the situation had been reversed? I hoped so. I found myself thinking how privileged we were to have had her care for Claire. The third apology came from the woman at the helm, the chief executive officer of the region. All three of these individuals understood that we cannot go back in time; we can only look back from where we are now. But they knew that the apologies were necessary so that everyone would be able to move forward.

Lessons to Learn

Nurses and physicians understand little about the grief of parents that follows the death of a child. Few have received any formal training in parental bereavement and in how to help those who are still living. In our case, the staff were completely overwhelmed with emotion, our and theirs, and felt it best to leave us alone — the safest option for anyone who really does not know what else to do. We need to do better.

The apologies meant a lot to us. But it has been the examination of what went wrong and how improvements can be made in the system that is more important. Vast changes have since occurred in the care delivered at the bedside in this particular PICU. Such changes always take time, patience and effort.

I wanted to share this story because I believe nurses, physicians and others involved in health care can learn from our experience. Those who truly care will want to understand what really matters to families on the other side of the locked door — and will want to do it better with the next child, with the next family.

Postscript

I am a nurse and a mom, also a wife and graduate student. I live in St. John's, Newfoundland and Labrador. Within the Eastern Regional Health Authority, I am known as "Claire's mom."

My daughter, Claire, died March 14, 2008, at the age of nine years at the Janeway Children's Health and Rehabilitation Center after a planned surgery and planned admission to the pediatric intensive care unit. Claire's death was not related to one simple event, but rather to the result of many lapses in care throughout her 16 days in the PICU.

She came through the surgery well. Even on the first day, however, there was a hint of the trouble to come when a chest x-ray showed the endotracheal tube (ETT) to be very high. The following day, a chest x-ray in the morning revealed collapse and consolidation of the right lung and the ETT still high. Later in the day, the collapse extended to the left lung and the ETT remained in its too-high position.

The cascade of events basically involved deterioration of Claire's lungs as the result of consistently high pressure on the ventilator, leading to acute respiratory distress syndrome (ARDS) and pneumonia. In ARDS, infections, injuries or other conditions cause the lung's capillaries to leak more fluid than normal into the air sacs. During this time, pediatric intensivists along with an emergency room physician covered the PICU. On day 4, following a decline in Claire's health and 12 days before her death, a PICU resident questioned the Full Code status without any discussion with us. When we became aware, and as the question continued to raise its head, we repeatedly confirmed the Full Code status. On day 11, we said, "No code if cardiac arrest." Following a discussion with physicians on day 15, Claire's status was changed to do not resuscitate. Claire died at 11 a.m. the following day.

At our request, Claire's care was reviewed from admission to autopsy by the Eastern Regional Integrated Health Authority. A team of reviewers from the ICU at Toronto's Hospital for Sick Children came to St. John's and, after a thorough investigation, Claire's death was determined to be "preventable" and accepted so by Eastern Health. From the review, we learned that the determination of code status had been done prematurely, there was a lack of knowledge on the part of all disciplines, and ventilator management fell below the standard expected of a tertiary-care PICU. There was a general lack of acknowledgement or acceptance of the external review findings by staff and physicians.

It has been quite a journey learning to accept and find our way, with all that we now know of the mistakes leading up to Claire's death, and that is further complicated by the fact that I do "get all sides." I worked in the same critical-care division in which Claire died. Those involved were colleagues, friends and friends of friends — quite a complex situation.

Following the external review, there was a buildup of both underlying and overt resentment by staff and physicians. Already strained professional relationships began to erode. The culture of "no blame" seemed to slide into a culture of "no accountability." Notable exceptions were those individuals at the administrative level.

Claire's story is extremely compelling, but very complex. I have been very careful as to how it is presented, as I have never wanted her to be used as a means of ridiculing the health-care system in general or Eastern Health here in Newfoundland and Labrador. For that reason, Claire's story has not reached the media, as I have been cautious. I made a choice to share her with certain groups and organizations first. And I made a choice to invite Eastern Health to do so with me as they needed to be part of the change.

After the external review, Eastern Health's CEO, vice-president, and director of Child Health and I put much effort into developing a PowerPoint presentation known as "Claire's Story." We have shared "Claire" regionally, provincially and at the national level through the Canadian Patient Safety Institute. Jointly, we looked at the "episode of care" and discussed the lessons learned as related to the processes of disclosure, apologies, family engagement, achieving accountability in a no-blame culture and barriers to changing clinical practice and culture. We also looked at the devastating impact of Claire's preventable death on us, her family, and also on the intensive care unit staff involved. I share "Claire's Story" from the perspective of a mom, a former critical-care nurse and an Eastern Health employee. It is impossible to separate the many hats I wear.

The apologies we received for the mistakes in Claire's care were not the expected "We are sorry Claire died" — I think that was definitely understood from the bedside to the boardroom in our situation. The apologies offered to us were more in line with "Claire died because of us — not in spite of us — and for that we are sorry."

Good people make mistakes. As a parent and a nurse, I have come to understand that we need to talk about those mistakes. But few health-care providers ever receive any formal training in how to talk candidly with the organization and with families and individuals when adverse events occur. When nurses, physicians and other health-care providers enter into the lives of patients and families, they become part of their story; we owe it to ourselves and to families to talk to them and each other when things go wrong or not as expected. Communication needs to occur from the top and the bottom.

Other lessons learned as we travelled the difficult road of getting answers to our difficult questions and then effecting change within the organization and the involved unit include:

- Blame-free cultures should not be allowed to translate into accountability-free.
- Disclosure and apology should be swift, sincere and all-encompassing and at all levels of the organization.
- Processes should be established and implemented for rapid response to concerns, external reviews and recommendations.
- Families should be given the information about what happened, how it happened and what is being done to ensure that it doesn't happen again.
- Honesty and openness are crucial.
- Each situation is unique; flexibility is essential.
- Ongoing discussions should be held with program staff and physicians.
- Challenging the status quo may be difficult but necessary.
- Working together with the family is much better than working around them.
- Outside consultants can provide support and help to effect change.
- Families should feel there is an acceptance of responsibility and accountability and steps are being taken to prevent a recurrence.
- Family-centred care is essential in diagnosis, treatment and outcome reviews.

We tell Claire's story simply with the hope of preventing a similar tragedy and with the hope of making the journey a little easier for the next family and organization that may travel in our footsteps. It has been a process in itself to get my head around sharing Claire's story and putting her "out there." I feel strongly that it has to be done in a certain manner, as Claire's death can't be just another sad story coming from our health-care system; there would be few next steps or lessons shared or remembered that way. The stories need to be shared. We are all responsible for safe and appropriate care.

This story is dedicated to nurses, doctors and health-care professionals who give their all each day to improve and save lives, and who feel humbled and privileged to be part of life and death, but most of all to Claire.

Extraordinary
People

On May 1, 2010, the Manitoba provincial government proclaimed the Personal Health Information Amendment Act (PHIA). Under the new amendment, current personal health information for patients and their families will be provided within 24 hours in hospital and 72 hours in personal-care homes and clinics, a significant shift from the former timeframe of 30 days. The amendment also states that institutions and physicians are required to inform patients of their right to authorize a family member or friend to access their health-care information.

The events that led to this amendment began on October 8, 2001, when Frances Raglan, 86, admitted herself to the Riverview Health Centre in Winnipeg for symptom relief from ankle ulcers. Following a rapid decline, she died 18 days later. During this time, nursing staff and management at the hospital repeatedly denied Frances's daughter, Mimi Raglan, access to her mother's health records. Privacy legislation was cited as the reason for denial.

Following their mother's death, Mimi and her siblings were provided with a copy of the medical chart. It was then they discovered that Frances had been placed on a care plan for the actively dying upon admission to the health centre. She also had been given a medication that she was not aware of and which had not been disclosed to or discussed with the family. Mimi contends that this medication contributed significantly to her mother's rapid demise. Mimi believes that if she had been allowed to see the medical records, she could have prevented her mother's death or, at the very least, been able to discuss treatment with her mother and care providers.

The initial decision by Mimi and her husband, Blake Taylor, to draw public attention to this issue evolved into a campaign to change the legislation the hospital cited to prevent access to Frances's records. This story tells of their dogged persistence over nine years and the help provided by Charles Cruden, Laurie Thompson and MLA Jon Gerrard that culminated in the proclamation of the PHIA amendment and the declaration by the Minister of Health, Theresa Oswald, that Mimi and Blake are "extraordinary people."

Diagnosis to Death: 1998 – October 26, 2001

Frances Raglan was a resilient woman who successfully beat the odds against ovarian cancer for more than three years. How much longer she would have continued to defy expectations had she received different treatment at Riverview is not known, but it could have been a matter of many months if not longer.

Frances was diagnosed with ovarian cancer in the spring of 1998. Following surgery, doctors said she had only a few months to live unless she underwent chemotherapy. She declined the treatment, instead relying on a healthy diet, nutritional supplements and daily exercise to maintain her health. Frances continued to live alone, eventually requiring some home-care assistance with meal preparation and bathing, until her October 2001 admission to Riverview. Although doing well by any standard, Frances knew she had a terminal disease and wanted to make responsible decisions regarding her future care. After a discussion with her family physician, she enrolled in the palliative care program at Riverview in April 2001. At the time, Frances was particularly interested in the home-care part of the program, which advertised ease of transfer to hospital for symptomatic relief of problems and transfer back home when symptoms were under control. As well, according to their publicity, the program included involvement of family in the planning of care.

In late June 2011, Frances went into hospital for control of diarrhea and sciatic pain. Within a week, she was doing well enough to go out on day passes. A couple of weeks later, she was discharged. During this admission, all of the program's promises were honoured. The attending physician was available, and Frances's family was included in the preparation of the care plan. Her symptoms were treated and she was sent home.

Anticipating a similar favourable experience, Frances requested admission in October for symptom relief of ankle ulcers, which were making mobility difficult. The care and attitude of nursing and medical staff and their relationship with the family, however, were in sharp contrast to the experience of her June admission.

To appreciate the full impact of the result of these changes, it should be recognized that in October 2001 there was no evidence that Frances was close to death. Indeed, she was healthy enough that the program's screening nurse did not think she needed to be admitted even for symptom relief. Mimi described the state of her mother's health: "My mother was in good condition. Her blood work had been stable for six months. A recurrent ovarian tumour continued to be documented as not painful. In fact, at the time of admission, the admitting physician wrote that he could not palpate any mass."

The unexpected cascade of events that followed caught both Frances and her family by surprise. They had little time and almost no information with which to understand what was happening let alone try to alter the course of events. They suspected something was wrong from the onset, and they had concerns about the attitude of nursing staff and patient-care managers, limited physician attendance, infections and pain control. Ultimately, Frances developed pneumonia and died.

Mimi described this time.

> Unfortunately, Frances had a new attending physician and some different nurses. My sister and I soon found that nursing staff, for the most part, now had a different attitude regarding the provision of care to our mother. Pain medications were frequently very late or nonexistent. Throughout Frances's ordeal, my sister and I tried unsuccessfully to find

out what was going on with our mother. She was deteriorating rapidly. She developed mouth, esophageal and bedsores. Later, she suffered a head injury and finally severe chest pains and pneumonia.

A week after Frances's admission, I spoke to the attending physician. I told him that my mother was getting worse, that her pain medications were frequently late or not administered and that no one seemed interested in helping her. He told me that if I had a complaint about care to take it to the health authority. Subsequently, he did arrange for a student nurse to attend Frances, for which she was grateful. The attending physician suggested that my sister and I stay home for a while, saying it was time to take a break. We did not take his advice.

On several occasions, we asked staff nurses and the patient-care manager to see our mother's health record and were refused. Privacy legislation was given as the reason. My mother's desire to involve me in care decisions was recorded in the nursing progress notes near the beginning of the admission.

Four days before her death, Frances suffered a fall resulting in head trauma. Contradictory accounts of the fall and the extent of injuries were given. Frances told Mimi and the attending physician that she had been dropped by two staff members and left on the floor beside her bed only to be eventually rescued by another staff member. She said there had been blood "everywhere" when she had been found, and it was "a huge job for staff to clean it up." When Mimi saw Frances the following morning, she had a bloody bandage on her head and there were blood stains on her pillow and large blood stains on her nightgown.

In subsequent conversations with the nursing staff, Mimi was told that her mother had apparently fallen on her way to the bathroom and there had been only a few drops of blood. She was told not to worry because the injury was minor. After filing a complaint and requesting the incident report, Mimi found confirmation that the injury was not minor. There was no mention in the report of Frances having been dropped by staff members. While her mother was alive, Mimi was not allowed to speak with the nurse who found Frances or any of the staff who were on duty the night of the fall. After Frances's death, Mimi was allowed to meet with the nurse who found her mother, and she confirmed that there had been a lot of blood as a result of the head injury. Mimi said:

> We found out that staff expected our mother was going to die only two days before her death. I left my mother's bedside briefly and when I returned, I found my sister crying in the washroom. She was accompanied by a nurse, the same nurse we had asked to be replaced because of her lack of interest in caring for my mother and because my mother found her intimidating. The nurse said to my sister and then to me, "Your mother's disease has progressed. I have talked to her and she is not afraid of dying and is ready to put herself in the hands of the Lord."
>
> At this point, the attending doctor came in and gave a quizzical look at the nurse and went to my mother's bedside. As soon as my mother saw him, she cried out, "Doctor, please help me! Save me. Save me!" He didn't say much of anything and soon left looking pretty uncomfortable! This whole episode might have taken 10 minutes. This plea for help by my mother was one of several she made to both nurses and doctors that went unheeded. By the day she died, it appeared that she had no trust in staff.
>
> In two earlier conversations, we had spoken to the attending physician about moving our mother to another hospital where she would receive better care. His response was "This [Riverview] is it." We asked about taking her home and were discouraged from doing so. The doctor said we would be on our own to care for her as they didn't have the resources. On the night before our mother died, we asked the attending doctor if he thought she would survive a transfer to another hospital, to which he emphatically said, "No." So we didn't move her. He subsequently said that we had refused an offer to have our mother transferred.
>
> Our family, including my brother who had flown in from Vancouver, was gathered around our mother on the day of the night she died. She was speaking to us occasionally, wasn't in pain and even asked for food. Later in the evening, a nurse injected a medication to help clear mother's congestion and asked us to join her in prayer. Approximately

45 minutes later, our mother abruptly stopped breathing. My brother, who had gone out for some supper, returned to find that our mother had died. A nurse offered her condolences to us and then abruptly asked if we could get our mother's things cleared out because the room would be needed in the morning.

Search for Answers and Accountability

After Frances's death, Mimi's brother, who was the executor of their mother's will, was able to obtain a copy of the health-care records. The family was shocked when they discovered that Frances had been immediately placed on a care plan for the actively dying upon her admission to Riverview. Mimi recalled:

> The documents clearly show that nursing staff had put my mother on a care plan for the dying right from admission, even checking off — falsely — that they had told our mother and us about their expectations on the day of admission. The palliative home-care coordinator did not make any notes at my mother's care plan meeting, meaning — as was later explained to us — that there had not been any plans for discharge. Subsequently, however, both the attending and prescribing physicians wrote in their letters to the College of Physicians and Surgeons that there had not been any expectation of my mother's death upon admission.

The second surprise for the family was discovering that Frances had been treated with a heavy course of a potent corticosteroid (dexamethasone) for 16 days up until her death. As well, they noted, there had been no plans to taper the dosage of this medication over time as is commonly done. Neither Frances nor her family had been aware that she was being treated with corticosteroids. Frances most certainly would not have agreed if she had known, according to Mimi. Her whole strategy, which had stood her in good stead for almost three and a half years, had been to support her immune system, not suppress it. It is Mimi's contention that her mother's severe oral and esophageal sores, much-worsened bedsores and pneumonia were likely a direct result of the immune-suppressing corticosteroid treatment or, at the very least, greatly exacerbated by the drug.

To substantiate her position, Mimi cited a paper, "Beauty Is Only Skin Deep: Prevalence of Dermatologic Disease in a Palliative Care Unit," authored by Dr. Cheryl Bernabé and Dr. Paul Daeninck, palliative physician and researcher for the Winnipeg Region Health Authority.[1] The authors stated that "aggressive use of corticosteroids is common." They further wrote: "Immunosuppression renders the patient more susceptible to opportunistic infections, causes atrophy of the skin and the underlying fatty tissue, decreases the protection available over bony prominences and increases the results of minor trauma. The proximal myopathy from prolonged use of corticosteroids contributes to immobility and thus predisposes to decubitus ulcer formation. Steroids also delay wound healing."

A university research scientist and professor of pharmacology who does analyses of drug regimens told Mimi and Blake that he could not pinpoint any reason that Frances was given the corticosteroid, but did say, "I'll warn you there are all kinds of ways they can justify using dexamethasone."

The physicians did give a variety of reasons for use of dexamethasone. In correspondence with Mimi, the attending physician wrote that dexamethasone is used in palliative care for a number of reasons, namely as a co-analgesic, an anti-nauseant to stimulate appetite, as an anti-inflammatory and for weakness. However, he did not specifically mention the reason(s) he used the drug as part of Frances's care.

The prescribing doctor had second thoughts about Frances's dexamethasone regimen. In a letter to the College of Physicians and Surgeons, the doctor wrote, "For someone as frail, compromised and elderly as Mrs. Raglan was, I would now start with a lower dose [of dexamethasone] and this concept I have gained with experience." The doctor added that "dexamethasone is usually started in a burst and subsequently tapered." In Frances's case, there were no orders to taper.

Over the next eight years, Mimi and Blake were in contact with various health and government agencies and officials. Not satisfied with the responses from Riverview, they approached the office of the provincial ombudsman and were told they should go back to Riverview with their concerns. The ombudsman's mandate at that time was primarily concerned with matters of administration by departments and agencies of the provincial or a municipal government. Several years later, changes were made, and the ombudsman had the authority to address Mimi and Blake's complaints under the Protection for Persons in Care Act (PPCA).

This legislation was enacted to help protect adults from abuse while receiving care in personal-care homes, hospitals or other designated health facilities. Under this law, the definition of abuse includes physical, sexual, mental, emotional and financial mistreatment. Any of these, alone or in combination, is considered abuse if the mistreatment is reasonably likely to cause death, serious harm or significant property loss.

Review of the Raglan case under the auspices of the Protection for Persons in Care Office (PPCO) resulted in nine recommendations for remedial action. These included ensuring that the care plan reflects the current health status of the patient and that the family is proactively involved. Also, it should be ensured that the level of pain is monitored and that medications are not only administered as ordered but also signed for when given. Mimi responded:

> These recommendations validated some of our concerns with care. However, the investigator did not investigate the appropriateness of medications given and found nothing amiss about staff's version of events about the fall. Despite the recommendations, the investigator found no fault with care. Our family was found to be sincere, but had insufficient evidence. Though we had been told that we would have another chance to speak with the investigator after her interviews with staff, we were not given this opportunity to refute the information she had been given at the hospital.
>
> We had initially received only a summary of the investigation report. We spent three years trying to get the complete report. Thanks to the efforts of the ombudsman, we did receive approximately 90 percent of it. The report was rife with provable inaccuracies about my mother's

health status and the care given, and even our family. For the most part, the evidence we provided was not addressed at all. In other instances, it was addressed with illogical explanations. I can certainly understand why they would not have wanted us to see it. This report has apparently been passed to other regulatory bodies to which we have appealed and has been used as an excuse not to investigate our concerns by health authorities.

We have pursued the problems associated with the report with the PPCO investigators, the former deputy minister of health and the current ombudsman with little satisfaction.

When Mimi and Blake contacted the vice-president of long-term care concerning comments he made regarding the PPCO report during a television interview, they were invited to meet with the VP and the chief patient safety officer of the Winnipeg Regional Health Authority. The two officials agreed with Mimi and Blake's request that they read their report on Frances's care in preparation for the meeting. It soon became obvious that the officials had neither read the report nor were they interested in its contents. Whenever Mimi tried to provide information, she was interrupted and told they weren't interested. The officials implied they had read the PPCO report, the bulk of which Mimi had not yet been allowed to see. In her words: "The meeting was short. I believe that they met with us only in order to say that they had investigated our concerns and found that there was nothing wrong with my mother's care, when, of course, there had been no such investigation."

In 2005, the new deputy minister of health met with Mimi and Blake. She was attentive, but later dismissed their concerns about Frances' care and the PPCO investigation and their request for an inquest. Mimi reported that the deputy minister did not answer their questions or address their evidence. However, the deputy minister did say publicly that changes were being considered to privacy legislation based on their concerns.

In 2007, Mimi, Blake and Dr. Jon Gerrard, a former palliative pediatric physician, MLA and leader of the provincial Liberal party, wrote to the College of Physicians and Surgeons concerning the appropriateness of Frances's care. The college investigator found that Frances had received standard care, but did acknowledge that the corticosteroid treatment "did not seem to do much good." The documented evidence Mimi and Blake submitted was not addressed by the investigator. Several requests to meet and discuss the documented evidence were refused. Gerrard wrote to the college suggesting it should issue a warning about indiscriminate use of corticosteroids, but says he has not received a reply.

The Personal Health Information Act and the Freedom of Information and Protection of Privacy Act

In addition to following the formal complaint processes required by various government agencies and regulatory bodies, as discussed above, Mimi and Blake simultaneously shared their concerns about the Personal Health Information Act (PHIA) with the community at large, primarily through the media. This approach eventually proved more successful. Mimi said:

> Knowing that the province's relatively new PHIA was cited as the justification for not giving our family the information we needed in order to help our mother with a crucial care decision, I thought this legislation and its implementation with its focus on confidentiality had greatly contributed to the problem. I also observed that its companion legislation, Freedom of Information and Protection of Privacy Act (FIPPA), was being used to prevent our family from seeing an investigative report that we had requested about our case.

As a first step, in October 2002, Mimi and Blake joined the Issues Committee of the Manitoba Society of Seniors (MSOS), an organization partially funded by the provincial government. Under the guidance of its chair, Chuck Cruden, Mimi and Blake convinced the committee to take up their cause. Subsequently, Mimi wrote an article for the MSOS journal about the problems with the PHIA and how it could be used to impede families trying to care for loved ones. This was the first of several articles on the topic they wrote for the journal over the next few years.

In early 2003, Chuck, Mimi and Blake devised a questionnaire regarding access to health-care information for readers of the MSOS journal. The large number of respondents were in almost complete agreement on the three questions: yes, people wanted to know about their right to choose an advocate who could access their records; yes, they wanted an advocate with these powers; and yes, they would prefer to have the information within 24 hours as opposed to 30 days.

Events in 2004 included a 12-minute feature by CBC Television on the Raglan story and problems with privacy legislation. Chuck, Mimi and Blake gave presentations to several public hearings during the review of PHIA and FIPPA. The *Winnipeg Free Press* began what would be a multi-year series of significant articles. Mimi recalled:

> We were very pleased to be receiving attention from our city's major newspaper as well as CBC Television, especially since we had already endured so many setbacks with our story being put on the back burner for two years. We had been disappointed on many occasions by another *Free Press* reporter who stalled and made excuses for not being able to write the article, and by a CBC Radio reporter, who had interviewed us, seemed very interested and then several months later withdrew without explanation. Later, we learned that her boss said that CBC had accepted the hospital's point of view that it was under no obligation to tell families anything. Our point that the Riverview Palliative Policy states that the families are to be included in the care plan apparently meant nothing to anyone except to Frances and our family.

In 2005, news articles about privacy laws in relation to Frances's case and the secrecy and delay over the PPCO report appeared in the *Free Press*. In one article and on CBC Radio, Deputy Minister of Health Arlene Wilgosh said she hoped there would be something in the upcoming mandatory Privacy Review of the Personal Health Information Act to address the Raglan family's concerns. Recalling that time, Mimi said, "We were very encouraged by these statements and the interest in improving privacy legislation, especially after she had refused to answer our questions about my mother's case."

Frances's family garnered a significant ally in fall 2005 when MLA Jon Gerrard decided to introduce their issues for discussion in the legislature and to the public on television. MLA Gerrard persisted in spite of often having to shout through the orchestrated heckling and theatrics from the government benches whenever he brought up various concerns regarding the Raglan case.

Early summer 2006 brought a huge blow to Mimi and Blake when they learned that only one of their recommendations to the provincial review of PHIA was included. This was an expanded list in hierarchical order of family and friends who could be included as a representative with the ability to access medical record information of an incompetent person. Although important, it was not seminal to their key concerns of a patient's right to authorize a family member (or friend) to have access to the information contained in their medical charts and be informed about this right as well as to have access to this information promptly. This was in spite of Deputy Minister Wilgosh's public statement that she hoped the recommendations would address their concerns.

Leah Janzen, a lead reporter for the *Winnipeg Free Press*, wrote an article about Mimi and Blake's disappointment with the PHIA recommendations, which appeared on the paper's Web Extra page. When Mimi asked why it did not appear in the printed newspaper or its electronic version, she was told by an editor that the topic was not of sufficient interest to the public.

In the fall of 2006, Mimi, Blake and Chuck joined the Winnipeg Regional Health Authority's Safety Advisory Council. By the end of the year, the committee had approved their recommendations for improved access to information for patients and families within the Winnipeg Regional Health Authority (WRHA). They were thrilled to learn that the WRHA board had given its approval as well. However, within a few months, the committee was disbanded and the policy changes abandoned. In the face of yet another disappointment, Mimi and Blake continued to speak out about the needs for changes.

In fall 2007, MLA Gerrard proposed a bill to give access to personal health information within 24 hours. The bill failed on second reading, but drew government attention to the issue.

The following February, the WRHA newsletter carried a statement that under new guidelines, hospital patients would be able to access their current care information within 24 hours. No one had contacted Chuck, Mimi or Blake with this news and they could not find any evidence of an updated policy on the subject. Mimi said:

> In May 2008, we were amazed to read in the *Winnipeg Free Press* that the PHIA would be amended and that patients would be able to see their records within 72 hours and that our other recommendations would also be included. We met privately with Health Minister Theresa Oswald twice. We also made presentations to the Provincial Legislative Committee after second reading of the bill, as did Chuck Cruden and Laurie Thompson from the Manitoba Institute for Patient Safety, whom Blake had successfully persuaded to support us. Blake and I, in debate with Heather McLaren, director of Manitoba Health's legislative unit, convinced the minister to change the time frame in hospitals to within 24 hours as well as to ensure that patients be made aware of their access rights including their right to authorize another person to access their information.

In October 2008, the PHIA amendment passed third reading and was given royal assent. Although acknowledgement was given in the legislature by all parties, there was no press coverage. Passage occurred late on a Friday afternoon, which is bad timing to attract the attention of the press. Mimi and Blake were disappointed at this anticlimactic nature of what they thought was the end of their long journey. What they didn't realize at the time, however, was that this was not the end. The bill had yet to receive official proclamation by the legislature. The proclamation occurred on May 1, 2010. The year and a half between passing third reading and proclamation was a busy time for Mimi and Blake.

They developed a video about their request to change the PHIA which includes news stories, comments by Minister Oswald and MLA Gerrard, volunteer safety advocates and representatives of the Manitoba Institute for Patient Safety. The video has been shown at national and international patient safety conferences.

They also worked with Minister Oswald's assistant on new information regarding patients' rights in the Manitoba InfoHealth Guide and a poster about changes to the PHIA. They assisted in the rewording of the WRHA's Access to Personal Information Policy. In spite of continuing frustrations, they persisted and were happy to see that the new guide included relevant information regarding patients' rights, informed consent and changes to access rights under PHIA. Thanks to their efforts, the new WRHA access and disclosure policies say that "current care" for personal-care homes is defined as three months rather than a week as originally proposed. This means that patients or their designates have access to medication lists, test results and progress notes for the previous quarter of a year.

Proclamation of the PHIA Act on May 1, 2010, elicited mixed feelings from Mimi and Blake. On one hand, they felt satisfaction in having been the driving force behind changing a provincial law, a considerable achievement by any standard. They had done what few other citizens have been able to achieve and in so doing honoured Frances by helping to ensure the safety of all patients in Manitoba. On the other hand, they have been disappointed at the lack of attention the amendment received from the media, especially outside the Winnipeg area. Around the time of proclamation, however, the bill generated some media coverage by the *Free Press* and CBC Radio.

Fortunately, under the new PHIA Amendment Act, information about the access to health information rights of patients must be prominently displayed in all Manitoba hospitals, clinics and personal-care homes. While the act is not yet universally applied, many of the major institutions are fulfilling the requirement and thereby helping to change the culture from secrecy to openness and partnership in care.

Mimi and Blake believe all patients in every part of Canada should be assured of the same access to their health information as is enjoyed by residents of Manitoba.

A Second Chance

Fervid Trimble, 87, enjoyed several additional years of quality life thanks to a caring and capable family who suspected a number of recently pre-scribed drugs might be responsible for her rapid cognitive decline. Following careful research by Fervid's daughter-in-law, Johanna Trimble, the family presented medical staff with their conclusions and the suggestion of a "drug holiday." Once off the recently prescribed drugs, Fervid returned to her former mental condition. Fervid died five years later following infection with antibiotic-resistant Clostridium difficile, *most likely acquired in the seniors' residence where she lived. Fervid's experience inspired Johanna to seek ways to help others, especially the frail elderly. At a patient safety conference a year after Fervid's death, she met a prominent advocate in the field who recommended she join a national patient safety group. Johanna now plays leading roles in patient safety groups at the national, provincial and local level. Working through the media and in public engagements, she educates the Canadian public about over-medication. In 2010, she won top prize at an international health conference for her poster, "Is Your Mom on Drugs?" She is currently involved in provincial programs to educate physicians about optimum prescribing practices and to assist frail elders to remain in their homes.*

In 2003, Fervid Trimble, 87, was admitted for a short stay to the health-care centre of the seniors' complex where she lived because of an unexplained spell of weakness and dizziness. For a number of years, she had lived in her own apartment in the complex and actively participated in life around her. Her only sign of mental decline was occasional forgetfulness.

Fervid's cognitive and physical abilities deteriorated rapidly in the health-care centre. Her worsening condition was not only of concern, but a source of puzzlement for her daughter Kathie, son Dale and his wife, Johanna, because the attending physicians were unable to diagnose the cause. The Trimble family began to suspect that at least some of the new drugs Fervid had been prescribed since admission to the health-care centre might be playing a role.

Aided by her background in library science, Johanna researched the new drugs, all of which had been prescribed without consultation with the family. She found that some were contraindicated and others not recommended to be given to the elderly. Others were known to be associated in various ways with causing serotonin syndrome. This syndrome is a potentially life-threatening adverse drug reaction that may occur following interactions between drugs.

Within weeks, Fervid developed seven of the 10 symptoms of serotonin syndrome, starting with changes in mental status, delusions and the inability to distinguish dreams from reality. She was agitated, lost coordination, displayed involuntary arm movements and had episodes of rapid heartbeat and sweating. She also had periods of unusual daytime sleep from which she was difficult to rouse.

Fervid's family met with the medical staff, presented the information Johanna had found and discussed their conclusions. The staff agreed to withhold the new drugs she had been prescribed. In the meantime, a psychiatrist for the care centre, who did not know Fervid's normal, healthy mental baseline, diagnosed her as having Alzheimer's and prescribed donepezil (Aricept). "We were flabbergasted! Mom had never shown any signs of Alzheimer's. We researched the risks versus benefits of the medication and declined to have her put on it. We also told the medical staff not to prescribe anything we had not previously approved," Johanna said.

The "drug holiday" restored Fervid's mental function to the level where she was able to participate in activities at the care centre. She also could join her family at her favourite seafood restaurant to dine on oysters and enjoy white wine when they visited.

Recalling this time, Johanna said: "This gave great joy to all of us. To our sorrow, though, she had lost considerable physical function from weeks of being bedridden. Had we known what we know now and been able to act sooner, she might have been able to return to an apartment, perhaps with an assisted-living arrangement, in the residence and to a more active life involving friends and social activities. This is an important consideration because of the debilitating effects that isolation may have in nursing-home settings."

In 2007, Fervid contracted antibiotic-resistant *Clostridium difficile*. This bacterium, which causes serious gastroenteritis, has a high mortality rate especially among the elderly and is often associated with institutions such as hospitals and long-term care facilities. Several other residents at the seniors' complex were infected with *C. difficile*. Johanna recalled that Fervid was not seriously ill and was given repeated doses of vancomycin, a powerful antibiotic. As Fervid's condition deteriorated, her family had difficulty in getting staff to give her the probiotics they brought and to ensure that she drank the rehydration fluids they supplied. Fervid also developed a stomach bleed, which the family attributed to warfarin (Coumadin) administered in dosages that were not properly adjusted to accommodate her dehydrated condition.

Fervid died at the age of 92 in October 2008 after sharing her philosophy and wisdom with her family: "Well, I think I'll leave all my love to the next generation. May they realize the agenda we've set out for them with love and affection. It's too precious not to live — we've enjoyed each other so much. I think it [love] will grow. That's the ticket into the next world. We will always be together, our love is always there and we will be part of the great growing field of love."

"If Mom had died in a confused and delusionary state four years earlier, we would not have received this gift of her wisdom, blessing and expression of love for her family," Johanna said. She, Dale and Kathie question to what degree the so-called epidemic of Alzheimer's and dementia is the result of over-medication. They encourage other families, caregivers and primary-care providers to consider over-medication as a cause for cognitive impairment, especially in the elderly.

Fervid's family is keen to share what they learned that may be of help to others.

- Listen carefully to your older family members and watch for new symptoms that don't make sense.
- Keep a detailed written record.
- Research and compare symptoms to drug side effects, especially when new drugs are suggested.
- Keep risk versus benefit in mind in the context of frailty, and consider the quality of life.
- When feasible, have family meetings, agree on your approach and let the coolest head in the family speak to those in authority.
- Bring your research findings and opinions to the attention of medical staff in a respectful yet persistent manner.
- Ask physicians to direct a trial to eliminate or reduce drugs.
- Request that family consent be obtained for any new drug(s).
- Debrief, console and support each other.

Johanna's background in library science and educational media was of considerable assistance when researching medications, their side effects and possible interactions. She found the five sources listed below to be particularly valuable.

- Therapeutics Initiative, University of British Columbia: www.ti.ubc.ca
- Public Citizen: Worst Pills, Best Pills: www.worstpills.org
- Cochrane Library: www.thecochranelibrary.com
- Dr. John Sloan's podcasts on the frail elderly (#76–78): therapeuticseducation.org/podcast
- Dr. John Sloan's *A Bitter Pill: How the Medical System Is Failing the Elderly* (2009) and his related website, www.sunshiners.ca

Following Fervid's death, Johanna asked herself how she could help make the medical system safer for everyone. She took courses and participated in workshops on how to be an effective advocate. In 2009, she attended the Empowered Patient Conference: Including the Patient in Patient Safety, held in Nanaimo, BC, and organized by Rhonda Nixon ("Forever Changed"). "I met Donna Davis ["Vance's Gift"] there and we spent three hours straight talking in the hotel room. She invited me to join Patients for Patient Safety," Johanna recalled. Today, Johanna is an active member of Patients for Patient Safety Canada, a working group of the Canadian Patient Safety Institute, the BC Patient Voices Network and the Vancouver Coastal Health Authority's Community Engagement Advisory Network. She recently received the designation of "Champion" from the World Alliance for Patient Safety (World Health Organization).

In October 2010, Johanna's poster, "Is Your Mom on Drugs?," won top prize in the category of teaching, treatment plans, protocols and cases at the Selling Sickness conference in Amsterdam. The conference, which attracted over 200 people from 20 countries, was hosted by *Gezonde Scepsis* (*Healthy Skepticism*, Netherlands). The Dutch Ministry of Health, the Dutch Health Care Inspectorate and the European office of the World Health Organization sponsored the gathering.

Educating the public about the dangers of over-medication is a priority for Johanna. She is a frequent participant in events related to medication and the elderly and also makes herself available to the media for interviews on health care and the frail elderly. Johanna was featured in the December 8, 2010, *Chatelaine* article "How Drug Reactions Can Be Fatal." The following year, Johanna was interviewed for the article "Is Your Mum on Drugs?," published in the August 24, 2011, issue of the *British Medical Journal*, and for "Too Many Pills," in the March 2011 Canadian edition of *Reader's Digest*.

Johanna spoke about some of her more recent activities.

My proudest moments have occurred recently. I want to change our health-care system at the level of care, not just attend meetings on systems and policy. To this end, I am a public member on the steering committee of a provincial initiative, the Optimal Prescribing Update and Support (OPUS) program, a continuing education project to update family doctors on best prescribing practices. This is an evidence-based antidote to the pharmaceutical companies' "detailing" where doctors receive much misinformation on drugs. We have presented our prototype session to "physician champions," who will then go out and teach other family doctors in BC through the recently formed Divisions of Family Practice. The divisions are community-based organizations of family doctors dedicated to addressing gaps in care in their particular communities.

I have also recently been involved in working with a team of medical professionals with whom I presented my mother-in-law's story of rescue from over-medication to a local group of long-term care professionals. Again, it is a prototype training session that will roll out provincially. We focus on presenting information on pharmaceuticals, methods of careful "de-prescribing" and the benefits in the context of frailty and quality of life. As geriatric specialists Mallery and Moorhouse of Dalhousie University pointed out in their article, "Respecting Frailty," published in November 2011 in the *Journal of Medical Ethics*, "Treatments may be offered without full consideration of the risks and benefits in the context of frailty. Health-care decisions may be made in response to a single issue, rather than considering overall health."

I am particularly excited about a recent invitation to act as a public member on a research team, including Dr. John Sloan, that is researching the benefits of treating frail elders in their homes with a 24/7 team-based approached involving the Home VIVE program of the Vancouver Coastal Health Authority. As well as being what most elders want, that is, staying in their homes as long as possible, the home-based team approach can prevent over- or inappropriate use of acute-care resources. Hospitals are not an optimal care setting for frail elders.

I also presented our story to almost 400 general practitioners and others in April 2012 at the 23rd Annual Drug Therapy Decision Making Course presented by the Therapeutics Education Collaborative of the University of British Columbia. The adversarial stance that many patient advocates are left with after an adverse event, and this includes myself, may be overcome by meeting and working with medical professionals. Many of these professionals are well aware of the problems and are working hard for change. I have been left with a positive response to my work as well as a feeling of mutual respect and acceptance as an important part of the "team."

PART II

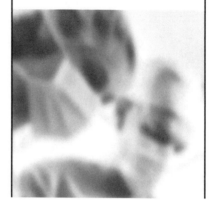

Whose Mistake?

Mark Handelman

Injury, suffering and death are some of the potential impacts of medical errors involving patients who were expected to live at the beginning of their treatment. But what is an error when death is anticipated to occur within hours, days, perhaps weeks? As discussed by Robert Sibbald and co-authors, including Mark Handelman, in their 2011 paper,[1] identifying errors at the end of life must take into account adverse outcomes other than death.

Not acting on prior capable wishes, not identifying legal substitute decision-makers (SDMs) and not explaining consequences of the treatment alternatives resulting in unrealistic expectations are examples of errors identified by Sibbald and colleagues. Allowing family members or SDMs to "direct" care resulting in treatment that is not indicated is another example.

Possible adverse outcomes of these errors include prolonged hospitalization and suffering for the dying person, confusion and tension between immediate health-care providers and the family and conflict between members of each of these groups. Psychological, emotional and moral distress may affect both family members and health professionals.

Several investigators have suggested that poor communication is a common thread among errors associated with end of life. So what can be done to avoid mistakes in communication at this difficult time? In this article, Mark discusses the roles of lawyers, health practitioners, patients and families in the prevention of errors associated with end-of-life communications.

Mark was called to the Ontario Bar in 1978. Currently, he is in the private practice of health-care law, representing health practitioners, SDMs and patients, and advising and teaching health-care providers. He is also a member of the Ontario Human Rights Tribunal and of the Society of Immigration Consultants' Discipline Tribunal. Mark was appointed to the Consent and Capacity Board of Ontario in 1998 and served in various capacities for 10 years. For a number of years, he was the board's only vice-chair for quality assurance and presided over approximately 2,000 board hearings, including the majority of the board's end-of-life cases.

Mark holds a master's of health science degree in bioethics and served as a member of the corporate ethics committees for both William Osler and Humber River Hospitals. He played a key role in the writing of the information brochure, "A Guide to Substitute Decision-Making." He has published widely on mental health law and ethics, substitute decision-making and the end-of-life process.

Introduction

In the autumn of 2010, Mr. Hassan Rasouli needed surgery to remove a tumour from his brain. Something went wrong, he contracted meningitis and ended up in what the intensive care specialists treating him post-surgery diagnosed as a persistent vegetative state. In the view of his treatment team, Mr. Rasouli would never recover and his best interests therefore dictated that he be allowed to die with dignity.

Mr. Rasouli's wife was his substitute decision-maker. She disagreed with the team, saying that his religious beliefs precluded anything less than taking all measures to keep him alive, even in a vegetative state. At this writing, the dispute between Mr. Rasouli's substitute decision-maker and his treatment team is heading to the Supreme Court of Canada, where the judges will have to determine who decides and perhaps how those decisions should be made.

Mr. Rasouli's case raises a variety of legal, moral, ethical and religious questions, only one of which is examined here: why didn't anyone know, before his surgery, what Mr. Rasouli would have wanted in the tragic circumstances following his surgery? It seems no one asked him and he didn't volunteer the information in advance of surgery.

Mr. Rasouli's situation is tragic but not unique: people simply do not like to talk about death and dying. Until about 1960, it didn't matter because the dying process would not be prolonged: your heart stopped and you died. We've changed that with technology that can do the work of the heart and lungs even after the brain has told those organs to shut down. The ventilator, as it is called in the vernacular, made open heart surgery possible and opened the door to organ transplants and innumerable other procedures that were previously impossible if not incomprehensible. Needless to say, this is all good.

But the ventilator has also made it possible to continue "life" long after the brain has shut down and rendered the euphemism "pulling the plug" a very literal question.

More to the point, when do you want your life support discontinued? Don't answer that question to me; answer it to the people who will be making that decision for you if the time ever comes that you cannot make it for yourself. And, as I think Mr. Rasouli's health-care team should have helped him do before surgery, make an informed decision about the treatments being proposed to you.

Informed Consent

For Capable Patients

You have the right to make an informed decision before consenting to any treatment and your doctor has the obligation to provide you with the available medical information relevant to that decision. Get that information, ask questions about it, understand and consider it before making a decision. Insist upon explanations of medical terms you don't understand and, when appropriate, take as much time as you need to make a decision. What you saw on prime-time television does not substitute for real information.

Many surgeons don't like to warn patients about worst possible scenarios; they want them confident of success, looking forward to their futures. A confident patient is easier to treat, easier to cure, more likely to recover. Except sometimes things do go wrong — ask Mr. Rasouli about that.

That point arose in the Court of Appeal, when one of the judges asked, essentially, "They were cutting through his skull to remove a tumour from his brain. Didn't anyone canvass what should be done if something went seriously wrong?"

Apparently not. One can speculate what happened: The surgeon explained the procedure, its benefits and *likely* risks. Mr. Rasouli knew he needed the surgery and the question of what to do if things went wrong was never raised. A few surgeons have explained to me that this is the common approach, and there's no need to caution patients about remotely possible worst case scenarios and leave them to worry about complications not likely to arise. Or the surgeon may have said, "There are always risks with any surgery, but I've done this procedure hundreds of times and never had a problem."

Is that informed consent? More precisely, is that the type of informed consent you want before surgery? If not, the obligation is yours to ask more questions.

For Incapable Patients

Who makes health-care decisions for a person unable to make his or her own choices? This is a legal question and the answer varies from province to province. Traditionally in such situations, the legal obligations rested with the attending physician to make decisions based upon the patient's "best interests." That remains the law in England and many Canadian provinces, though English courts have recognized that if the decision will likely result in death and there is any question or dispute about what is appropriate, the physician should make a court application to determine the question.

The more modern approach is for legislation to create a hierarchy of substitute decision-makers (SDMs) whose responsibility it is to give or refuse consent to treatment. In Ontario, for example, the Health Care Consent Act has such a hierarchy. At the top of it is a court-appointed guardian of the person if the guardianship order authorizes that person to make the decision. Next comes the patient's attorney for personal care, if there is a valid power of attorney for personal care appointing one or more attorneys. Next comes the patient's spouse, partner or parent.

The Ontario legislation also sets out the principles upon which such decisions must be made. I can make a foolish decision about my own treatments but, as an SDM, my obligation is to make treatment decisions for the incapable person based upon his or her previously expressed capable wishes applicable to the circumstances. If there are no such wishes, my decision must be made based upon the person's "best interests," a defined term that not only includes the objective medical factors but also considers the patient's values and beliefs.

The two most common problems arising in treatment decisions for incapable patients at end of life arise when the SDM holds out hope for a recovery that the health practitioners deem unrealistic or when the SDM does not know what the patient would have done for himself were he able to make the choice.

The Lawyer's Mistakes

Most jurisdictions in the English-speaking world now allow a person to write an "advance care directive," though they are called different things in different places. In Ontario, for example, the Substitute Decisions Act authorizes a person to write a power of attorney for personal care, a POA (PC), a document that names the attorneys and sets out any wishes relevant to treatment decisions. "No heroic measures" provisions are common.

A common scenario is the client who wants a will and powers of attorney. Hours will be spent deciding who to name as executors, which child will get the silverware and dishes, which charities to make contributions to and how to minimize taxes at death. Part of the financial planning package includes a power of attorney for property, but the POA (PC) is often an afterthought.

Lawyers need to not only explain the significant of a POA (PC) but also how to ensure it works as intended.

The person or persons you name as your attorney for personal care may well have to make life and death decisions on your behalf. The most common decision will be when active treatment should be discontinued because palliative care is appropriate — in the vernacular, when to pull your plug. Lawyers must bring home this fact to their clients. The client might make his or her own foolish decision, but it should at least be informed.

If you tell your lawyers you want to name all three of your children as your attorneys, did he or she ask how they get along? Adult children who still fight over who gets the cottage on a particular weekend and cannot resolve such a question civilly are unlikely to agree upon *your* correct end-of-life decisions.

Few lawyers encourage clients to talk to the people they're thinking of appointing to make their health-care decisions. Has your lawyer helped you pick an attorney or attorneys who understand your values and beliefs and who have the courage to advocate on your behalf with health-care professionals and to give or refuse consent to treatment decisions based upon your values and beliefs rather than their own?

Has your lawyer insisted you talk to your proposed attorneys, first to ensure they are willing to accept the responsibility and second to empower them to make the difficult decisions as you want them to be made? And finally, has your lawyer suggested you choose someone with the courage to advocate for you at all stages of your treatment?

A Short Checklist for Lawyers

- Did you explain the importance of a POA (PC) to your client?
- Did you help the client determine whom to name as attorneys for personal care?
- Did you explain *every provision* in the document to your client?
- Did you make sure your client talked to the proposed attorneys to ensure they are comfortable with the obligations this role imposes and to ensure the attorneys will respect the client's values and beliefs — and have the courage to implement them?

The Doctor's Mistakes

A person admitted to hospital with broken bones is likely to have a visit from a dietician if someone thinks he or she is significantly overweight. Smokers get visits from hospital staff who encourage nicotine replacement therapy. If your home is a shambles that could put your health at risk, you receive a visit from a discharge planner to ensure safe transition from hospital back to community.

However, few hospitals and almost no doctors offer advice of any sort on the end-of-life decision-making process unless your medical condition is imminently terminal.

Doctors may or may not understand the legal processes in place to assess a patient's capacity to make his or her own decisions, understand the definition of "capacity" to make treatment decisions or the hierarchy of substitute decision-makers and the principles upon which substitute decisions must be made.

Physicians may also not be clear in communicating to either patients or their families about the patient's condition and prognosis or take the time to answer the myriad questions that arise when treatment decisions are final. They sometimes (even unintentionally) revert to jargon. The answer to the following question is unlikely in most cases to meet the test of informed consent: "As a result of CVA, your husband suffered anoxic brain injury and is now PVS. We'd like to palliate him, okay?"

A Short Checklist for Health Practitioners

- Did you assess the patient's capacity to make his or her own treatment decisions and chart your findings?
- Did you ask if your patient has a POA (PC), or has otherwise identified the correct SDMs? Did you place a copy of the document in the patient's chart?
- Did you enquire about the patient's values and beliefs pertaining to his or her own end-of-life decisions?
- Did you explain the patient's condition and prognosis to the SDMs

in terms they could understand and take the time to answer their
questions?

* If the SDMs are making what you consider to be a bad treatment
decision, did you explain your hospital's dispute resolution process
and (in Ontario) the role of the Consent and Capacity Board in
resolving disputes between decision-makers and treatment team?

One case in particular stands out in my mind. The patient, in his
late 8os, had end-stage dementia. He was unable to speak and barely
aware of his environment, with no prospect of recovery. His bedsores
were extensive and his body could no longer heal them. He suffered
repeated bouts of pneumonia, received nutrition through a feeding
tube inserted directly into his stomach through an incision in his
abdomen and could not breathe without the assistance of a ventilator.

This man's wife insisted "everything be done" to keep him alive;
that this is what he would want because he was a religious man who
saw the sanctity of life as being above all other factors, who would have
wanted to suffer if that was what was necessary to prolong the fight.
What astonished me about all of this is that end-stage dementia is not
a condition that suddenly appears: Dementia takes years to develop
and symptoms usually become apparent before the victim loses his or
her capacity to capably express end-stage treatment preferences. But,
throughout the entire course of this man's illness, including months
in hospital, it seems no one canvassed his views on the end of his own
life.

The Patient's Mistakes

Go through the checklists for lawyers and doctors and pick up any
stray pieces they've missed: At the end of the day, your health care
and your treatment decisions remain your responsibility!

Do you have a power of attorney for personal care? Have you
named responsible people to make decisions for you when you cannot?
And have you talked to your future substitute decision-makers, first to
tell them your end-of-life wishes, second to ensure they will seek to

achieve them and third to ensure you have bestowed upon them the courage and certainty of mind to achieve your end-of-life goals?

Have you read your power of attorney, just to ensure it says what you want? Many lawyers insert a "no heroic measures" provision, expecting that is what the client wants, but does it accurately reflect your views?

When the decisions remain yours because you are still capable, will you make informed decisions? Will you make sure you understand the treatment your physician proposes, asking for explanations of medical terms you don't understand?

No Heroic Measures?

What does that even mean? The answer is, it means different things to different people and different things at different times. Some doctors will tell you that, given the strides in medicine over the past half century, there are no longer any heroic measures, only expensive ones. Others will tell you that what might be considered heroic today will be commonplace in a decade or less.

Your end-of-life decisions should be less concerned with a particular treatment than with your prospects for recovery from what ails you and the quality of life that will follow.

When my mother was in her mid-80s, she needed surgery for bowel cancer. We went together to meet the surgeon and he did a thorough job of explaining the risks and benefits of surgery. Mother understood and consented, but there was one more issue: The doctor explained that sometimes as part of surgery, resuscitation is required and Mother was the subject of a "do not resuscitate" directive.

Mother didn't remember she'd agreed to a DNR, if she ever did agree. And it was a blanket DNR, which did not address her circumstances at the time she needed resuscitation. Suppose she'd tripped in her kitchen and knocked herself out, should she be resuscitated? I would certainly hope so. Needless to say, we rescinded the DNR. And by the way, the surgery was successful, she lived almost another decade and had the good fortune to die asleep in her own bed at the age of 94.

I've given considerable thought to my own end-of-life wishes, spent time explaining them to those who will make the decisions for me if I am incapable and encapsulated my thoughts in my own Power of Attorney as follows:

> Death is as much a reality as birth, growth, maturity and old age. It is the one certainty of life. I recognize this. Therefore, while I am incapable, should a situation arise where my attending physician determines that I will not recover from a disability and that my death is imminent, I DIRECT MY ATTORNEY to permit me the dignity of a peaceful passing. I do not wish to be kept alive by measures that would only serve to prolong my dying process, but I rather wish to die with dignity and in comfort. In that situation, I wish for treatments that will allow me to die peacefully even though they may abbreviate the dying process, resulting in a hastening of my death.

Most important, I spent time talking to the people who may have to make these decision for me, first to make sure they would be willing to assume the responsibility, second to ensure they understood what I meant by what I wrote and third to empower them to respect my wishes.

Children: A Special Case

In Ontario, there is no minimum age at which a person is entitled to make his or her own health-care decisions. Children, if capable, are entitled to decide for themselves. In other provinces, the concept of "the mature minor" is gaining traction, with a bit of a push from the Supreme Court of Canada in a recent case.

But parents think they know best for their children and want to make their decisions, especially when they involve life and death issues.

How can we balance the child's right of self-determination against parents who want what they think is best for the child? In my opinion, the balance comes with a clear understanding on the part of parents and the child's treatment team of what it means to be "capable" with respect to the decision. Assessing a young person's capacity to make an important medical decision can be very difficult, requiring far more probing questions than with an adult.

But another aspect is this: Parents called upon to make substitute decisions for children usually do so based on their own beliefs and not those of the child. Very young children simply do not have a system of values and beliefs and their decisions should be made based upon more objective best-interests considerations. A two-year-old simply does not believe in God.

How and When Do We Talk About Death?

Death isn't anyone's favourite subject. But, difficult as it is to broach, it is important.

Opportunities, however, do arise. People die on television all the time and it isn't too hard to broach the subject between the end of a medical television show and the start of the nightly news.

When my mother was in her early 80s, she called me one day to ask if I could take her to the funeral of a close friend. Mother and I talked about her own end-of-life views on the way home from the funeral. She raised the subject for the first time, upset that her friend had to linger through the dying process while her family decided what to do. So I asked her for her own views. It was an easy segue.

Mother was not an educated person, but she was certainly wise and able to sum up her own views pithily and succinctly. She told me, "When there's nobody home, you turn out the lights, don't you?" I knew what she meant and I shared the story with my sisters, but we were fortunate enough to be able to avoid the decision for her.

Conclusion

The process of informed decision-making rests upon communication between the health practitioner and either the patient or the patient's substitute decision-maker. Simply put, a person making health-care decisions needs to understand the risks and benefits of a proposed treatment (including worst possible scenarios) and the alternative treatments.

Substitute decision-makers need to understand the wishes, values and beliefs an incapable patient's decision would have been based upon. Neither a person's autonomy nor the concept of "patient-centred care" will work without that understanding.

The Media

Susan McIver

As shown in the stories in this book, the media is a key component of health-care advocacy. In this section information is presented on how to use the media effectively.

Newspapers, magazines, radio and television are powerful tools of communication. These traditional means efficiently deliver content to a large number of people. They do not, however, allow for participation in the creation or development of the content in the same way as the rapidly evolving area of social media. There are a variety of types of social media, ranging from social sharing sites such as YouTube and Flickr through social networks such as LinkedIn and Facebook. A wide range of technologies are also used, for example, websites, instant messaging and emails.

Social media allows for the unregulated dissemination of information within a network or community of individuals with similar interests. The danger is that potentially libellous material or simply an unfair representation of events that occurred can be posted. In traditional media, good reporters and editors check for accuracy and potentially libellous material. Whichever means of communication you use will depend on your goal, the message and the target audience.

Other factors include available time to do regular updates of social media sites, technical expertise and the degree of privacy desired.

The Basics

Regardless of how your information is delivered, there are two basic rules. You must thoroughly know your subject and be prepared to back up everything you say. (See Investigative Tip System at page 215.) Obtain a copy of your medical records and have a qualified friend or associate help you to interpret them. It may be helpful to hire your own medical expert to review and report on your situation. As well, you should learn about and know how to navigate the systems relevant to your situation — hospital, health regions, provincial laws, professional college policies. Be sure to address recommendations or complaints to the appropriate regulatory body.

The second rule is to always have your emotions under control. This is especially true if you are being interviewed shortly after a devastating event. It is crucial that you are emotionally and psychologically strong enough to handle the exposure and to answer tough questions that may be asked. Going to the media before you are ready can harm your story. There is little point in being "just another sad story." If you are upset, you are also more likely to say something you will later regret, such as laying blame and making accusations rather than focusing on what needs to be changed.

Be polite and professional when dealing with newspaper reporters and radio and TV hosts. For the most part, media people are well intentioned and may be sympathetic to your situation. An important part of their job, however, is to provide balanced coverage by showing all sides of a situation. Don't be surprised if someone with a different point of view is also interviewed or if you are asked to respond to what your critics would say. Don't get angry. Remember to tell journalists only what you want in your story. Nothing is ever completely "off the record."

Your Goals and How to Achieve Them

Knowing your goals is important in selecting the means of communication and achieving success in delivering your message. Do you want to make contact with others who have had a similar experience? Do you want hospital policies and procedures changed? Do you want attitudes changed? Do you want to educate the public? Do you want to educate certain medical specialists? Do you want the laws governing the health-care system changed? Your goals may change over time. Express your goals clearly, whether you are posting on Facebook or speaking with a reporter.

In some situations, the media may come to you, such as during or at the end of an inquest or if the circumstances of a death are particularly newsworthy. If you are prepared and in control of yourself, welcome the opportunity to inform the public about your specific situation or issues. A particularly good time for you to approach the media is on the release of a coroner's or other official report. This type of non-biased information adds significant credibility to your story. Other times to contact the media include when launching or settling a lawsuit, even an out-of-court settlement, and when a coroner's recommendation has been put into place. Let the media know about your activities. Have you established an organization? Given a public presentation, organized a conference or spoken to a group of health professionals?

Health care is one of the hottest topics in the news. Journalists are looking for good, reliable, well-researched stories to personalize their reports. It's almost always easy to approach and work with the media. Here are some useful suggestions.

- *Contact:* Telephone or email the editor of the local paper or a reporter who specializes in health issues or a radio or TV announcer. This approach works best in smaller jurisdictions; however, reporters for large papers are also always keen to find good stories. Explain the key points of your case and what you hope to achieve. Be concise. Newsrooms are busy places.
- *Media release:* A media release is one page long and begins

with a headline written in bold. In the first paragraph, state who the story is about, what is happening, where and when it is happening and why the issue is important. In the next few paragraphs, explain clearly why your story needs to be told and provide further information and quotes from key people. Put your contact information on the last line. If you have particularly pertinent additional material, such as figures, quotes and a summary of previous media coverage, include these on a second page.

- Protect yourself against libellous comments. Stating an opinion is not libellous, but making a definitive statement you can't prove in court could be. To state your opinion, start a sentence with "in my opinion," "I feel," or "I think." Use this approach when giving interviews as well as writing media releases.

- Make a list of the relevant local, regional and national media. The internet is an excellent resource to help you find where releases and stories should be sent. Check your local bookstore and newsstand.

- Follow-up phone calls to editors or journalists are important. Did they receive the media release? Do they have questions? Again, be brief but do use the opportunity to pitch your story again. As an example, you might say "the recommended changes will save lives."

- Be persistent. Sometimes the decision to use a story is not made until the next day or later at a story meeting. Keep a log of your calls, the names of the people to whom you spoke and the outcome. Be prepared to call back.

- *Provide visuals:* Photos or videos from before the medical mishap humanize your story and help readers or viewers relate to what happened and what you want to accomplish. Have copies of the photo or videos ready for the media. Even the most conscientious journalist may be unable to return the material to you.

- *Doing an interview:*
  - Be prepared and answer questions directly and briefly. This is particularly important for live interviews, because there is no opportunity for editing.

- Have notes handy when doing telephone interviews for radio and newspaper reporters. Don't read from your notes, but have them ready in case you go blank.
- If a reporter calls you by surprise and you are not prepared, ask for a few minutes to get your notes and collect your thoughts or ask the reporter or announcer to call back in a few minutes.
- TV interviews require more preparation. First, be sure to wear the same type of clothes as the TV journalist. This will help give you credibility with viewers. Second, memorize a brief line that captures the essence of your message. Such "clips" or "sound bites" will likely go on air unedited.
- When an interview is about to end and you haven't had the opportunity to mention something crucial, politely ask if you can mention an important point.
- *Difficult questions:*
    - If an interviewer tries to get more information from you than you are comfortable giving, simply repeat your initial response until he or she realizes you are in control and moves onto the next question.
    - If an interviewer asks a question that you think is inappropriate, you can remain silent or say that you had a different understanding of what the interview was about. This approach is preferable to saying "no comment," which will be aired or printed, and then you will be seen as having refused to answer and possibly as being contentious. If you remain silent, there is a chance the question will be deleted from the article or program.
- *Corrections:* On occasion the media can get the story wrong or opponents will say things that aren't fair or true. Immediately contact the editor or producer with corrections or a rebuttal. If an expert has been misquoted or comments misconstrued, get his or her support when approaching the media outlet. You may succeed not only in helping to provide accurate information, but also possibly in generating more stories about your case.

- *Media conferences:* Media conferences are held to announce particularly significant information and can be held by anyone.
  - Seek advice from publicists, activists and anyone else with experience.
  - Be thoroughly prepared.
  - Send a carefully prepared announcement to the media.
  - Select your time and location carefully.
  - Sometimes individuals and groups can hold media conferences in city or provincial government buildings free of charge.
  - Additional speakers, such as medical experts and opposition politicians, give the conference a boost.
  - Talks should be no longer than five minutes to allow for time for questions from the media.
  - Use visuals to illustrate and emphasize your message.

The media, whether traditional or in the evolving area of social media, is a powerful and essential tool for effecting changes in health care.

Investigative Tip System

Gordon Nixon

Gordon Nixon was a Royal Canadian Mounted Police officer for 26 years. During part of this time, he served in the general investigation section where he employed the investigative tip system in various types of investigations, including homicides. The chapter "Forever Changed" is the story of his wife Rhonda Nixon's work in patient advocacy following a surgical error.

The investigative tip system was a method of keeping and organizing records that police used in complex investigations before the advent of suitable computer programs. The goal of the system was to take a large amount of information from a wide variety of sources and break it down into easily understood portions. These in turn could be collated and cross-referenced into succinct and supportable conclusions.

The tip system can be of considerable assistance to lay people who may not be sure if, in fact, an error occurred or, if it did, may have difficulty in grasping its complexity. A simple inquiry to the relevant administrator or health-care provider may resolve the matter. If concern persists, formal complaints can be lodged with appropriate oversight organizations and professional colleges or associations. Other avenues can be explored, such as obtaining the opinion of an independent medical expert or seeking legal advice. Keeping detailed records of every action is the key to formulating and substantiating concerns.

The first step is to obtain all records associated with every aspect of the situation. These records may include police, autopsy and coroners' reports in addition to medical records kept by hospitals, in doctors' offices and anywhere else treatment and diagnostic procedures have occurred. Individuals are entitled to obtain copies of their medical records and records of relatives for whom they have medical power of attorney or equivalent designation. There may be a charge associated with photocopying the records.

Medical records are a complex set of documents that may be hundreds, perhaps even thousands, of pages in length. Depending on the case, these may include doctors' orders and progress notes, admission forms, diagnostic laboratory reports, emergency room forms, nursing notes, medication records, care plans, surgical and anesthesia reports, consent forms, vital sign sheets, do not resuscitate orders, bowel care records, ambulance reports and discharge summaries. These are rarely provided in a well-organized, collated manner.

Ideally, all medical records will be in the documents provided by the hospital. Make sure they are. Read all reports and records carefully. Ask a friend or an acquaintance, such as a nurse, nurse practitioner or physician, for help in collating complex medical records and understanding the medical terminology and procedures. If applicable, consult two or more knowledgeable people.

Request your medical records in writing. Keep a copy of every request in a separate file which will eventually also contain responses. The first requests should go to the hospital, family physician and any specialists. Make requests as broad as possible, using language like "and any other documents related to my care." Depending on circumstances, it may be necessary to request copies of relevant policies and procedures. If the information provided is incomplete, make additional written requests itemizing what may be missing. Retain the original copies of all records and replies in a secure location. Make as many working copies as necessary.

Keep the records from each source in their own file for easy reference. Collate the records by date so that you can create a time-line of care. The timeline becomes its own file, as do other facets of the case. If multiple packages of records are received, make sure each package is placed in its own file. Record the date of receipt for each package, a summary of its contents and how it differs from the others. Each doctor involved in a case will have most likely been given the same report or laboratory result; however, examine each document closely, as often the physician will have made handwritten notes which may provide valuable insight into the situation.

The way my wife, Rhonda Nixon, and I organized the investigation into her case illustrates how to use the tip system. We found a banker's box, the "tip box," convenient for storing files. In Rhonda's case, she had seven specific complaints and numerous concerns about her care which formed the basis for her complaints to two different medical bodies. The files were:

1. Complaint to the College of Physicians and Surgeons of British Columbia
2. Complaint to Vancouver Island Health Authority
3. Complaint 1
4. Complaint 2
5. Complaint 3
6. Complaint 4
7. Complaint 5
8. Complaint 6
9. Complaint 7
10. Additional concerns
11. Albumin transfusion record
12. Prescription summaries
13. Disability claim
14. Medical records from Doctor "A" (general physician)
15. Medical records from Doctor "B" (surgeon)
16. Medical records from Home and Community Care Nursing Services
17. Medical Services Plan billing records
18. Report from Doctor "C" (chiropractor)

19. Records from physiotherapist "D"
20. Records from registered massage therapist "E"
21. Informed consent policy of hospital
22. Consent Practice Standard for Registered Nurses and Nurse Practitioners
23. PubMed article related to patient's care
24. PubMed article: "ERCP Related Perforations: Risk Factors and Management"
25. *Physician's News Digest* article: "Effect of Medical Error Disclosure and Apology"
26. SpringerLink article: "Survey of Informed Consent of Endoscopic Retrograde Cholangiopancreatography"
27. Surgeonsblog, January 31, 2007, complications and bile duct injuries, written by Doctor "F"

Attachments

- Six discs of imaging received from hospital
- Copy of first set of medical records received from hospital
- Copy of second set of medical records received from hospital

Each of the above files contained specific information which assisted in proving the complaint or clarifying statements. It is important to clearly state the complaint at the top of the file, for instance: "Complaint 1 — Doctor 'A' failed to disclose," and summarize what the doctor failed to disclose. Some documents were relevant to several different files or alleged complaints. In those situations, a separate copy of the document was included in each file or complaint.

The first file summarized Rhonda's complaint and provided copies of documents used to identify those physicians included in the complaint and to illustrate key facets of the case for the College of Physicians and Surgeons. Likewise, the second file contained a relevant summary of the complaint to the health authority and documents related to that complaint. Files 3 to 9 each dealt with a specific complaint and contained relevant supporting documents.

Some of the files contained more than 20 pages of summary and attached documents. The file identified as "additional concerns" detailed over 30 specific issues, such as inaccurate charting, incorrect names of treating physicians, inaccurate billing records and failure to provide complete and accurate medical records.

Rhonda provided copies of all documents (files 10 to 28), imaging discs and hospital records to each agency conducting a review of her complaint. This meant that each of these agencies had the same information Rhonda had used to reach the conclusion which formed the basis of her complaints. She also included related articles to illustrate her concerns and provide context for reviewers. Reports from health-care professionals involved in Rhonda's recovery and subsequent ongoing care provided context to the extent of her injuries. They also showed the risk in which other professionals were placed because of the non-disclosure of the original error.

In Rhonda's case, the billing records from British Columbia's Medical Service Plan (MSP) confirmed the dates and costs of all treatments provided in or out of hospital. Billing records in other jurisdictions can be equally useful. MSP and similar records can reveal treatments not otherwise disclosed. The dates on these records help to corroborate dates of key events which may be in dispute. These records also contain the name of the physician who performed a procedure. In Rhonda's case, there was an error regarding the name of a surgeon in the hospital's records.

Finally, it is extremely important for patients and their advocates to keep a personal detailed record of care. Such a record or journal provides an account outside of the "official" medical record. Be sure to note dates, times, names of doctors and nurses involved in care, medications provided, tests performed, issues of cleanliness and any related points of care. As previously mentioned, complex medical cases can generate hundreds of pages of non-collated medical records. A journal can be crucial in organizing events and highlighting significant points. A journal may also be the only way to keep track of care while in hospital. Customarily, hospitals do not release medical records until a patient has been discharged.

Medical
Malpractice
John McKiggan

Should I consult a lawyer? That is a question often asked by patients and families affected by medical errors; yet, as studies have shown, most do not. In this article, John McKiggan, QC, a founding partner of Arnold Pizzo McKiggan in Halifax, provides information to help individuals and their families better understand the medical malpractice claims process. Equipped with such information, patients and families can make a more informed decision about whether or not to pursue a medical malpractice claim.

John's father and grandfather were respected physicians in Nova Scotia and he anticipated following in the family's medical tradition. John earned a science degree in biology and anatomy and was preparing for medical school when he began to have second thoughts. He realized that most of the qualities shared by great doctors — compassion, understanding, honesty, humanity, competence, commitment, empathy, respect, creativity and a sense of justice — were also traits shared by great lawyers. And so he went to law school. He has dedicated his practice to providing peace of mind to people who have been seriously injured through medical malpractice, auto accidents or institutional liability. He has a special interest in representing survivors of childhood sexual abuse.

John's colleagues have honoured his efforts and experience by electing him president of the Atlantic Provinces Trial Lawyers Association. He has been appointed Queen's Counsel (QC), a designation used to recognize

Canadian lawyers for exceptional merit and contribution to the legal profession. John was selected by his peers for inclusion in The Best Lawyers in Canada 2012 in the field of personal injury law.

John is a frequent contributor and presenter at legal conferences throughout Canada and internationally. He is also an accomplished writer. John was nominated for an award of exemplary journalism covering issues related to the sexual exploitation of children by Beyond Borders ECPAT Canada, a national non-profit organization that advances the rights of children to be free from sexual exploitation. He was nominated in the print category for his article published in the Lawyers Weekly: "The Catholic Church and Sexual Abuse: Is the Church's Response Real Action or Window Dress?"

What is Medical Malpractice?[1]

Medical malpractice is the term typically used by lawyers to describe negligence by a doctor. But medical malpractice can involve negligence by other health-care providers, including nurses, chiropractors, ambulance attendants and paramedics, or hospital staff, such as x-ray technicians and lab personnel. Perhaps the easiest way to define medical malpractice is: "Substandard care from a health-care provider or institution that causes injury or death."

Medical malpractice can happen in many ways:

- If your doctor did not have your *informed consent* to perform a medical procedure that caused you an injury (more about what informed consent is later in this chapter).
- If your health-care provider was negligent, and the negligence caused an injury or death.
- Medical malpractice can also be caused by an institution (like a hospital) not having proper equipment to treat patients or proper policies and procedures in place to protect patients against injury.

How Often Does Medical Malpractice Happen?

Because medical malpractice can involve negligence by a variety of different health-care professionals or institutions, it is surprisingly difficult to find exact statistics about how often medical malpractice happens. What information we do have likely vastly underestimates the incidence of actual medical malpractice occurrences in Canada.

A famous study by Harvard Medical School determined that over half of all injuries caused by medical mismanagement (in other words, not caused by the patient's initial injury or disease) were preventable, and another quarter of those incidents were caused by negligence.

In a different study, researchers at Harvard determined that only 2 percent of people injured by negligence actually made a malpractice claim.

A reported published in the May 25, 2004, edition of the *Canadian Medical Association Journal* entitled "The Canadian Adverse Events Study: The Incidence of Adverse Events in Hospital Patients in Canada" confirmed findings of similar studies in the United States, Australia, the United Kingdom, Denmark and New Zealand.

"The Canadian Adverse Events Study" concluded:

- As many as 24,000 patients die each year in acute care hospitals due to "adverse events" (doctors' term for a bad result or a mistake).
- 87,500 patients admitted annually to Canadian acute care hospitals experience an adverse event.
- 37 percent of adverse events are "highly" preventable.
- 24 percent of preventable adverse events are in relation to medical errors.

Every preventable medical error or adverse event is a potential medical malpractice claim. So according to the Canadian Medical Association, more than 100,000 potential medical malpractice claims happen in Canadian hospitals every year. That doesn't include mistakes by chiropractors, paramedics and other health-care providers. In short, the figure of 100,000 potential malpractice claims is just the tip of a very large iceberg. Medical mistakes have an impact on thousands upon thousands of Canadians every year, most of whom never know they have been a victim of potential malpractice.

A report by the Canadian Institute for Health Information (CIHI) indicated that nearly one quarter of Canadian adults (that's 5.2 million people) reported that they, or a member of their family, had experienced a "preventable adverse event," in other words, a medical error.

Role of the CMPA

In Canada, most doctors are defended by a single organization, the Canadian Medical Protection Association (CMPA).

According to their 2010 annual statement, the CMPA had $2.69 billion dollars in assets (money in the bank). The CMPA uses this money to hire the best experts and lawyers money can buy to defend doctors who are accused of medical malpractice.

Many victims of serious medical errors cannot work, or they have huge expenses for ongoing rehabilitation and medical care. Against such overwhelming financial odds, Canadian victims of medical malpractice face huge challenges to obtain justice and fair compensation for their injuries.

Remember that there are over 100,000 potential medical malpractice claims in Canada every year. During the five-year period from 2005 to 2010, the CMPA reported only 4,524 lawsuits were filed against doctors in Canada: fewer than 1,000 claims per year. Out of more than 100,000 potential medical practice victims, 99 percent never filed a lawsuit!

The CMPA is proud of its success rate in defending claims brought against doctors. During the same five-year period, 3,089 claims were dismissed or abandoned because the court dismissed the claim or the victim or the victim's family quit, ran out of money or died before trial.

Some Frightening Statistics

- Of 521 cases that went to trial, only 116 resulted in a verdict for the plaintiff. In other words, of the few cases that made it all the way to trial, only 22 percent of malpractice victims actually won their trial.

- For the plaintiffs who won at trial, the median damage award was just $117,000.
- Of more than 4,000 lawsuits filed against doctors from 2005 to 2010, only 2 percent resulted in trial verdicts for the victim.

In other words, 98 percent of potential Canadian medical malpractice victims never received a penny in compensation!

Are Canadian Medical Malpractice Claims Different than in the United States?

In a word: yes. But perhaps not in the way many people would think.

Lots of people have read about large jury awards for personal injury claims in the United States. Sometimes American jury awards seem to be out of proportion to the injury.

In Canada, court awards are usually much lower than awards for similar injuries from courts in the United States. Cases that might be successful in the U.S. are simply not economically feasible to pursue in Canada.

But the biggest reason medical malpractice claims are more difficult in Canada is because of the role the CMPA plays in defending doctors.

In the United States, most doctors have medical malpractice insurance provided by companies like the insurance company that insures your car or house. These insurance companies are publically traded and they have to make profits for their shareholders.

If an American malpractice insurer has a claim worth a million dollars that it can settle for $500,000, it makes financial sense to do so. It saves money for the company and is good for shareholders.

Similarly, if an insurer is defending a small claim that may be expensive to fight, it makes financial sense to pay something to settle the claim to avoid the increased cost of litigation. This is what insurance companies refer to as a nuisance settlement.

The CMPA is *not* an insurance company and is not intended to make a profit for members. The sole reason for the existence of the CMPA is to defend doctors accused of misconduct and it does so vigorously without consideration of cost.

For example, the CMPA will not settle a claim simply because it costs more to defend than the claim is worth. The CMPA can afford to spend $200,000 to fight a claim that's worth only $25,000. With its enormous financial resources, the CMPA can afford to spend whatever it takes to defend doctors accused of malpractice.

What most Canadians do not know is that the provinces and various medical associations have negotiated arrangements that require government to reimburse doctors for some of their CMPA dues (or similar medical liability insurance premiums).

Reimbursement programs vary depending on the province. Currently, Saskatchewan pays 1 percent of doctors' CMPA premiums. In Ontario, the province pays 80 percent. This amounts to hundreds of millions of dollars across the country every year.

In BC, a 2008 media report stated the province paid doctors $22 million to reimburse them for CMPA premiums. The same year, a Freedom of Information request revealed that Ontario taxpayers spent $112 million to subsidize CMPA dues. Doctors paid $24 million.

Dues vary by practice specialty with the high-risk specialties paying more. The current annual CMPA fee for an obstetrician in Ontario is approximately $86,000. But the province pays almost the entire premium. Doctors pay just $4,900 of the $86,000 premium.

In 2009, the CMPA spent $76 million dollars on legal fees defending doctors in lawsuits across Canada. It comes as quite a shock to the injured malpractice victims that I represent when they learn that their tax dollars are being used to defend the doctors who may have injured them.

The Burden of Proof in Medical Malpractice Cases

When something goes terribly wrong after medical treatment, it is human nature to look for someone to blame or to assume that the bad result was due to negligence. But in many cases, the bad result is just that; a bad result that happened even when the patient received competent and reasonable care. So in every medical malpractice claim, the plaintiff bears the burden of proving their case.

Most people have heard the term "proof beyond a reasonable doubt." That is not the burden that applies in medical malpractice claims; it is the burden that applies to criminal trials.

In a medical malpractice claim, the plaintiff must prove their case "on the balance of probabilities." In other words, is it *more likely than not* the doctor was negligent *and* that the negligence caused your injury?

The easiest way to think about this is to consider a pair of scales. All the evidence for your claim is placed on one side of the scale. All the evidence against your claim is placed on the other side of the scale.

As long as the scales tip to the side for your claim, even a little bit, then you have met the burden of proof on the balance of probabilities.

What Do I Have to Prove to Win My Medical Malpractice Case?

Generally speaking there are two ways to win a medical malpractice claim:

1. Prove that your health-care provider didn't have your "informed consent" to perform the medical procedure that caused your injury; or
2. Prove that your health-care provider was "negligent" and that the negligence caused your injury.

What Is "Informed Consent"?

Every adult has the legal right to decide what can be done with his or her own body. This is called autonomy. Because of this legal right, doctors need your permission (the legal term is consent) before they can treat you.

Sometimes doctors or other health-care professionals are found to have been negligent because they did not get the patient's "informed consent" to the medical procedure.

You can only give valid permission if you are provided with all the information necessary to make an informed decision about the proposed medical treatment.

For example, it is not acceptable for your doctor to simply ask your permission to perform surgery on your leg.

You must be able to understand why the surgery on your leg is necessary and the reasonable and foreseeable consequences of giving your permission (consent), or not giving permission, for the surgery.

It is generally accepted that in order for you to provide proper permission ("informed consent") for medical treatment, your doctor must explain:

- The nature of the proposed medical procedure;
- The reasonable alternatives to the proposed medical procedure; and
- The relevant risks, benefits and uncertainties related to the procedure and each alternative.

Any medical procedure that is performed without informed consent is considered to be an assault. The person who performs the medical procedure will be responsible for any injury you suffer as a result of the procedure.

Unfortunately, it is difficult to win medical malpractice cases based on lack of informed consent. In cases where the plaintiff's version of events differs from chart notes, or consent forms, courts tend to prefer the written records.

Sometimes there are no written notes, charts or records about what risks were explained to the patient. The question of whether the risks were properly explained to the patient boils down to the doctor's word against the patient's.

In most of the reported medical malpractice decisions across Canada, judges and juries tend to favour the doctor's word, unless there is clear evidence to support the patient's version of events.

It is important for patients to document the consent process by making notes of any discussions you have with your doctor before you undergo a medical procedure, particularly any discussion about the risks, benefits and alternatives of the medical procedure.

What Is "Negligence"?

Doctors and nurses are human. They are not expected to be perfect. But they are expected to perform their jobs to the standard of a reasonably competent doctor or nurse. If they fail to meet that standard, that's negligence. Negligence is defined as a failure to meet the standard of a reasonable person.

What does that mean in a medical malpractice claim? There are four things that every medical malpractice victim must prove to receive compensation for their injuries:

1. The standard of care.
2. A breach of the standard.
3. The breach caused an injury.
4. The damages (harm) from the injury.

Standard of Care

In a medical malpractice claim, you will need to provide evidence to show what the standard of care is in your particular case. Usually this requires your lawyer to retain a doctor (or doctors) in the same specialty as the negligent doctor who is willing to testify what the standard is and how the conduct of the doctor fell below accepted standards.

The standard of care may be different depending on who provides the medical care or where you are treated.

Medical specialists are held to a higher standard than family doctors. Courts expect specialist who have received additional training to be able to diagnose and treat illnesses and conditions that family physicians might not have the expertise to diagnose and treat.

Where the negligence happens may make a difference to the standard of care. For example, a doctor practising medicine in a rural hospital that does not have access to an MRI machine or other sophisticated medical equipment may not be held to the same standard as a doctor practising in a teaching hospital in Vancouver, Montreal, Toronto or Halifax.

Breach of the Standard

You will need expert evidence to prove that the health-care provider did not meet the standard expected of a reasonably competent professional with similar training and experience.

In other words, did they do something that they should not have done, or did they fail to do something that they should have done?

Causation

You must also prove that the failure to meet the standard of care (the breach) is what caused your injury.

A doctor's care may fail to meet accepted standards, but the failure may have nothing to do with the patient's injury.

For example, not wearing surgical gloves during an operation is a breach of the standard of a competent doctor. But failing to wear surgical gloves isn't likely to cause a patient to suffer a stroke during an operation.

On the other hand, failing to wear gloves may contribute to a surgical wound becoming infected, leading to serious injury or death.

Proving causation is usually the greatest hurdle patients face in medical malpractice claims. The medical and scientific issues surrounding causation are complicated and hotly contested in every claim.

Damages

Money can't replace the loss of a loved one or truly compensate for a catastrophic injury. But the courts try to provide a fair and reasonable measure of financial compensation to victims who have been injured as a result of the negligence of others.

The goal of a judge or jury in any personal injury claim is to try to put the injured person (or their surviving family members) in the same position they would have been in if the negligent act had not occurred.

Non-Pecuniary Damages

A non-pecuniary claim is one that does not result in a direct, out-of-pocket financial loss but is still considered to be worthy of compensation. Non-pecuniary damages are commonly referred to as compensation for "pain and suffering" but they cover all non-financial losses.

How Do the Courts Calculate "Pain and Suffering"?

There is no such thing as a "pain-o-meter." An injured victim cannot be hooked up to a machine that prints out the financial value of their pain. What judges or juries do in determining compensation for pain and suffering is use their experience and discretion to consider how the victim's injuries have affected their life and limited their ability to function.

Canada's Cap on Compensation for "Pain and Suffering"

In 1978, in a case known as *Teno v. Arnold*, the Supreme Court of Canada created a barrier to recovery for victims who have been injured as a result of someone else's negligence.

In the *Teno* case, the Supreme Court ruled that no matter how seriously injured you are, the maximum compensation you can receive for what is commonly referred to as "pain and suffering" is $100,000.

Taking inflation into account, the cap on pain and suffering awards is currently considered to be about $350,000. But the maximum amount is only paid to the most catastrophically injured victims (quadriplegia, severe brain damage and similar injuries).

If someone who must live in a wheelchair for the rest of their life because they are quadriplegic can only receive $350,000, what should a malpractice victim receive for a less catastrophic, but still serious injury, say the loss of a leg?

Most injured victims who are successful receive compensation awards that are far less than the (current) "maximum" of about $350,000. Remember, according to the CMPA statistics, the median damage award in malpractice cases is only about $117,000.

Fatal Injuries

There is no way to truly place a value on the loss of a loved one due to a fatal injury. In fatality claims, courts provide compensation for "loss of care, guidance and companionship."

Holding hands with your spouse, seeing your child graduate, asking your parent for advice — what are these worth in dollars and cents? As the credit card commercials tell us, these experiences are priceless. How do the courts determine a value that accurately compensates for the loss?

The honest answer is that they do not. Courts in Canada do not put a price, or attempt to calculate, the sorrow or grief we feel over the loss of a family member.

How much surviving family members are entitled to receive depends a great deal on the facts of each case. The courts in each province have established nominal ranges of compensation they will award to family members.

Many of us have read news reports of cases in the United States where surviving family members have been awarded huge sums of money for the death of a family member. The laws in Canada regarding compensation for fatal injuries are very different, and compensation awards rarely reach the levels seen in American cases.

Pecuniary Damages

A pecuniary claim is one that has resulted (or will result) in a direct out-of-pocket financial loss. For example, the cost of paying for medical treatment is a pecuniary loss. Past and future incomes loss is also a pecuniary loss.

Income Loss

Your injuries may cause you to miss a great deal of time from work. Perhaps you may never be able to work again. The courts will try to reimburse you for the loss of your income.

There are two elements to any loss of income claim:

- Past loss of income: You are entitled to be compensated for your actual income loss up to the date of settlement or trial. Usually this loss is one that is capable of being calculated fairly accurately.
- Future loss of income and pension benefits: There is no such thing as a crystal ball. No one knows for sure what will happen in the future. But if it is likely that your injuries prevent you from being able to work in the future, you are entitled to be compensated for that loss.

Diminished Capacity

Your physical abilities, your education, training and experience are all assets that allow you to earn an income. If any or all of those abilities have been limited or reduced to some extent by your injuries, you may be entitled to compensation for diminished capacity.

Valuable Services

If your injuries prevent you from being able to perform a physical chore or activity you normally did before you were injured, the court may compensate you for the financial cost of hiring someone to perform that valuable service.

For example, I have had many clients whose injuries have prevented them from being able to perform their normal housekeeping chores. We have made claims to compensate for the expense of hiring housekeepers to come into their home to do laundry, wash their dishes, make their beds. I have had clients recover compensation for the cost of mowing their lawn, shovelling their sidewalk and generally maintaining their home. I represented a single mom who suffered a spinal cord injury and was confined to a wheelchair. We were able to recover compensation for her for the cost of hiring a childcare worker to come into her home to help care for her two young children until she was able to care for her children on her own.

Sometimes other family members perform extra chores or duties that they would not otherwise have had to do if their family member hadn't been the victim of medical malpractice. For example, I helped parents recover compensation for the extra work involved in caring for a brain-injured child. Obviously, as a family member, we want to help the ones we love and don't expect to be compensated. But the courts recognize the extraordinary efforts that go into caring for a catastrophically injured family member. Courts can compensate family members for the valuable services they provide in caring for their loved one.

Cost of Medical and Rehabilitative Care

People who have been seriously injured often have significant ongoing medical expenses for physiotherapy, massage therapy, chiropractic treatment, medication, in-home nursing care and so on.

In the case of catastrophic injuries, the lifetime cost of ongoing medical care can be enormous. In one medical malpractice case, we represented the family of a child who had been seriously brain injured. The cost of providing medical care to the child was calculated by our experts to be $2,113,373.

Why 98 Percent of Potential Malpractice Victims Receive No Compensation

Tens of thousands of Canadians every year are victims of medical errors that could lead to a potential medical malpractice claim. But only a small fraction of Canadians ever receive compensation for their injuries. There are a number of reasons why patients do not recover compensation for injuries suffered while receiving medical care. Most of these reasons stem from general misconceptions about medical malpractice.

They Just Don't Know

Patients don't know they are victims of medical malpractice. In Canada, roughly 7.5 percent of admitted hospital patients suffer some sort of medical error or "adverse event." Canadian hospitals have documented over 100,000 "adverse events" annually. But according to CMPA annual reports in the past 10 years, the number of lawsuits against doctors in Canada has dropped "dramatically" by almost 50 percent.

Most health-care professions have ethical codes of conduct that encourage disclosure of medical errors to patients. But, incredibly, most provinces do not have any laws that impose a legal obligation to tell patients they have suffered a medical error nor any penalty for failing to do so.

In the vast majority of medical malpractice cases, injured patients and their family members simply have no idea that a poor medical outcome may have been caused by malpractice because no one tells them and they are too shocked or grief stricken to ask.

Loser Pays

In Canada, we have what is known as a "loser pays" rule. In most cases, the person who loses a lawsuit has to pay some of the legal fees and all the out-of-pocket expenses of the person who wins the lawsuit.

The theory behind the "loser pays" rule is that if you know you will have to pay the defendant's legal expenses if you lose, you will think twice before filing a lawsuit that doesn't have merit. It's hard to argue with that.

But the "loser pays" rule has the unintended effect of discouraging people with legitimate lawsuits from pursuing their claims.

Assume you have been seriously injured as a result of medical malpractice. You can't work, your bills are piling up and you can't pay your mortgage. Your lawyer tells you that if you file a lawsuit and lose, you may have to pay the defendant doctor or hospital tens of thousands of dollars. What are the chances that you are going to proceed with your lawsuit?

I have had dozens of cases over the years where the medical evidence indicated the patient's injuries were the result of medical malpractice. But the patient decided not to pursue a medical malpractice claim because if they lost the lawsuit, they might be ordered to pay legal costs to the doctor they accused of malpractice.

No Autopsy

In fatality claims, family members have the burden of proving the doctor's negligence caused the patient's death. Sometimes the cause of death is obvious. But in many cases it is impossible to prove the death occurred because of malpractice, because no autopsy was done to establish the cause of death.

Value of the Claim

We decline dozens of cases a year where it appears the doctor was negligent, but the resulting injury is not significant enough to justify the enormous cost and expense of a malpractice trial.

For example, we reviewed one case where the patient was given the wrong medication and had a serious allergic reaction. He was violently ill for almost two weeks. He lost time from work as a result. But he had a good recovery.

Even though we thought we could prove the doctor was negligent in prescribing the wrong medication, we determined the client didn't have a claim that was economically worth pursuing. The costs of the case would likely be greater than the expected recovery.

Statute of Limitations

Each province has its own time limit, called a statute of limitations, for filing a medical malpractice suit. The length of time may be different in each province, and the time when the statute starts to run varies as well. A statute of limitations can begin to run when medical services are rendered, when an injury is discovered (or should have been discovered), or some combination of the two.

If the time limit to file a claim runs out before the patient files their claim, their right to receive compensation may be barred forever.

Experts

You cannot win a medical malpractice case without one or more very qualified medical experts. They can be hard to find. It is becoming increasingly difficult to find doctors who are willing to stand up for what's right. It takes time and money to find the best experts for your case.

In 2009, the CMPA spent $12 million dollars to hire medical experts to defend doctors in malpractice claims. This is one area where the CMPA has a tremendous advantage. They have a "stable" of experienced medical experts they can call upon to defend doctors accused of malpractice. Most patients cannot afford to have several experts look at their case in order to find the one that will give them the "best" answer.

Common Defences in Malpractice Claims

The most common defence in medical malpractice claims is either a denial that the defendant was negligent, or a denial that the negligence, if there was any, caused the plaintiff any injury.

But there are a number of other creative defences that are commonly raised in medical malpractice claims.

Unexpected Injury

The injury was an unforeseeable consequence of the medical treatment. For example, one client we helped suffered serious injuries as a result of side effects from medication given to him by his doctor. The doctor argued the side effects were so rare that they were not foreseeable.

It Was the Patient's Fault

The injury was caused by the patient not following medical advice. For example, in one case we reviewed the patient didn't attend his appointment for a chest x-ray and eventually died from undiagnosed lung cancer.

It Was Someone Else's Fault

Someone else was responsible for causing the injury. In one case we successfully settled, the doctor argued that the hospital's faulty medical equipment, not the doctor's negligent care, was responsible for my client's serious brain injury.

The Patient Knew the Risk

The patient's particular injury was a recognized risk of the procedure and the risk was properly explained to the patient. In other words, the patient gave informed consent to undergo the risks of the procedure.

Pre-existing Injury

The injury was caused by a previous illness or disease. For example, the doctor may claim that your disabling back pain was not the result of negligent surgery but due to pre-existing arthritis.

Tasks in a "Typical" Medical Malpractice Claim

Medical malpractice claims often take years to settle or get to trial. Sometimes it is difficult for the client to understand what is going on behind the scenes during the process. The following list includes most of the significant tasks that have to be completed during a medical malpractice claim.

- Interview the client and family members;
- Educate the client about medical malpractice claims;
- Gather evidence including medical records and hospital documents;
- Interview potential witnesses;
- Determine if there are reasonable grounds to pursue a medical malpractice claim;
- Collect other evidence, such as photographs of the injury itself;
- Research all the legal issues, such as contributory negligence and informed consent;
- Review all of the client's relevant medical charts and records;
- Talk to the client's doctors or obtain reports to fully understand the nature of the client's injuries;
- Review the client's insurance policy to see if any money they spent to pay the client's bills must be repaid;
- Determine if the client must reimburse any insurance companies,

social assistance plans or employers for any benefits they may have paid the client;

- Read relevant medical literature to determine if malpractice was involved in the client's injury;
- Make recommendations regarding settlement;
- Find and retain medical or nursing experts to review the client's claim and provide a medical-legal opinion;
- Draft the Notice of Claim identifying the legal issues involved in the claim;
- Prepare the client, witnesses and medical providers for discovery examinations;
- Prepare written questions and answers for the defendants or their experts;
- Conduct the discovery examination of the defendant and other witnesses;
- Provide the defendant with all relevant information about the client's claim, like medical bills, medical records and tax returns;
- Ask the court to set trial dates;
- Prepare for trial and/or settlement before trial;
- Prepare for and conduct mediation hearing to try to settle the claim;
- Prepare the client and witnesses for trial;
- Organize and prepare medical exhibits for trial;
- Organize and prepare demonstrative exhibits for trial;
- File legal briefs and motions with the court;
- Take the case to trial with a jury or judge;
- Analyze the jury's verdict or judge's decision to determine if there are grounds for appeal.

How Do I Find a Qualified Medical Malpractice Lawyer?

Choosing a lawyer to represent you in a medical malpractice claim is an important but daunting task. There are certain things you can look for that will help lead you to the best lawyers for your case — no matter what type of claim you have.

Referral: Get a referral from a lawyer that you know and trust. Most of my medical malpractice cases come from referrals from other lawyers or satisfied clients.

Respect: Has the lawyer earned the respect of his or her peers? In most provinces, lawyers who are recognized as having made significant contributions to the legal community are awarded the honorary title of QC (Queen's Counsel). There are directories like *Best Lawyers* or the *Canadian Legal Lexpert Directory* where lawyers rate the abilities of their peers. Being recognized and included in these directories is a good indication of the respect the lawyer has within the legal community.

Experience: Experience is a big factor in most cases. Simply put, the more experience a lawyer has, the better the chances of getting a favourable result.

Books or Publications: Ask the lawyer if they have published books about their area of practice. This is a good indication of the lawyer's knowledge and experience. Ask if the lawyer has written articles for publication at legal conferences or academic journals.

Teaching Others: Does the lawyer teach other lawyers in continuing legal education courses? Lawyers who are recognized as having particular training or expertise in their fields are often called upon to teach or train others lawyers.

Moving Forward: Improving Canada's Health Care System

Silence Isn't Golden

Unfortunately when a doctor, nurse or other health professional makes a mistake, the tendency has been to hide the mistake and drop the "cone of silence" in fear that if a patient is told a mistake was made in their care, they will be more likely to file a lawsuit.

In actual fact, the exact opposite has happened. For example, in 2001, the University of Michigan Health System adopted a mandatory policy of disclosing medical errors and offering apologies. As a result, the number of malpractice lawsuits filed against the hospital dropped by a stunning 65 percent.

Most people who contact a medical malpractice lawyer, at least in my experience, are not looking to sue anyone. They are usually frustrated by the wall of silence they face from their doctor or the hospital when they try to get answers to their questions.

Safe to Say "I'm Sorry"

In the past, health-care providers have been reluctant to apologize to patients for their mistakes. The fear is that an apology may be taken as an admission of legal responsibility for the patient's injuries.

Four provinces in Canada have adopted (and others are considering) "apology" legislation to protect persons who make an apology from potential civil liability. The legislation states that any form of apology:

- Is not an admission of fault or liability;
- Cannot be considered by a court when determining fault or liability; and
- Is not admissible in court as evidence of fault or liability.

Saying "I'm sorry" can mean different things depending on the circumstances and can have very different results in the medical-legal context. This type of legislative initiative should be carefully considered.

For example, "I'm sorry your mother didn't survive the operation" offers sympathy but doesn't indicate legal responsibility. The statement provides comfort and closure to the family.

"I'm sorry I wasn't able to save your mother" may be interpreted as an admission of personal responsibility, depending on the circumstances.

"I'm sorry I killed your mother" appears to clearly contain an admission of fault.

Doctors shouldn't face the possibility of litigation because they offered sympathy to patients or grieving family members. But should they be protected if they clearly acknowledge and admit their fault?

Do Medical Malpractice Claims Improve Patient Safety?

Aside from being a means of providing compensation to victims who have been injured by medical negligence, do medical malpractice claims serve a larger purpose in society?

By holding defendants accountable for negligent misconduct, and forcing them to change their behaviour, our tort system helps make society safer.

For example, in the 1980s, the American Society of Anaesthesiologists was facing discontent from members as a result of increasing insurance premiums and negative publicity from medical reports of malpractice cases. The society conducted a review of closed malpractice claims. The information was used to create guidelines to improve patient safety. The result was a massive decrease in adverse events and deaths associated with the use of anesthesia.

Perhaps the most well-known Canadian example is how medical malpractice claims arising from tainted blood transfusions eventually resulted in a federal investigation (the Krever Inquiry).

Final Thoughts

The contributors to this book are truly inspiring individuals. At the outset of this project, we knew we would meet dedicated people who use their time, talents and financial resources to make health care safer. However, we discovered the contributors to be more than dedicated. In the past three years, we have come to appreciate their courage, their outstanding achievements and their heroism. We have also come to know and learn about physicians, nurses, other health-care professionals and lawyers who, through their association with the contributors and through their own work, are striving to improve patient safety. We thank the contributors for the honour of allowing us to tell their stories in the hope that others may not only recognize their achievements but also realize that they too can help create a better world.

The day my late daughter, Katherine Eileen Hallisy, was diagnosed with cancer, I knew my life was forever changed. What I didn't anticipate was that her illness would take me down a path that has led me to more than a decade of patient safety and advocacy efforts.

My experiences are intertwined in some way with the themes of every story in this book. The accounts in *After the Error* are from Canadian families, but they reflect the universality of medical harm. Their stories are all of our stories.

Every person who falls victim to medical error faces disbelief, isolation and despair. We are often told that we are the cause of the problem — we are too sick, too old, we didn't seek help soon enough or we didn't communicate our questions or needs effectively. At some point, each of us felt forsaken by the very system that we always believed would be there in our time of need.

My daughter was infected with *Staphylococcus aureus* while in the operating room for a "routine" 30-minute biopsy procedure. Already coping with the horrors of dealing with metastatic cancer, we were immediately engulfed by the formidable and unforeseen enemies of medical error and hospital-acquired infection. As Kate was rushed to the pediatric intensive care unit and placed on life support, I naturally assumed that we had yet again come out on the losing side of our health battles.

The doctors told us that our daughter's sudden illness was a rare and extraordinary event, and we believed them. The reality was that Kate's infection was not diagnosed correctly or treated properly for several days, which lead to septic shock resulting in permanent lung and kidney damage. After speaking with other parents at the hospital whose children were harmed by hospital infections, we started to have doubts. Then, in 1999, the Institute of Medicine released a groundbreaking report about the challenges and dangers in the American health-care system. The IOM report gave credence to the experiences of so many of us by stating publicly that medical errors are both common and often completely preventable. Medical harm is now seen as a worldwide epidemic and the solutions will involve a global effort.

As this book illustrates so well, many people who become patient advocates simply do not accept the status quo, which is that delivering medical care in a complex environment inevitably leads to high levels of harm. We believe that the voice of one person, against all odds, can make a real difference. And when that one voice is added to the sustained efforts of others who share our journey, the world can change.

Solutions that patient advocates were told were impractical, or even impossible, are now seen as innovative. Every time the powers that be say it can't be done, we question their explanations and challenge their complacency. We cannot, and will not, stop pressing for a better way. We want to validate our own experiences, to honor our loved ones and to show others that there is no need for them to learn our tragic lessons the hard way. It is our consolation, and our dream, that our pain will lead to positive outcomes for others.

In the United States, we see health-care improvements that are the direct result of consumer activism — including public reporting of errors, accessibility to medical records and calls for safer medical devices. Patient advocates raise awareness with efforts such as the creation of reference and educational materials for patients, websites, blogs and social media campaigns. We work with established consumer advocacy organizations and we create our own groups to move patient issues forward. Patients sit on family advisory councils, hospital committees and government groups. These changes may have seemed impossible in the not-so-distant past, but they are clearly our future.

After the Error illustrates the choices that individual citizens made to channel their negative experiences into positive action. The patient voice, so long excluded from improvement efforts, is now seen as the key to meaningful progress in building health-care systems that are safe, effective and compassionate.

Julia Hallisy, B.S., D.D.S.
San Francisco, California
Founder and President
The Empowered Patient Coalition

Introduction

1. Institute of Medicine. 1999. *To Err Is Human: Building a Safer Health Care System.* Washington, D.C.: National Academy Press.
2. Wolters Kluwer Health. 2012. "Nearly One in Three Americans Report Experiencing Medical Mistakes, Either Themselves or Among Family and Friends." Available at wolterskluwerhealth.com. News archives, August 15.
3. Landrigan, C.P. et al. 2010. "Temporal Trends in Rates of Patient Harm Resulting from Medical Care." *New England Journal of Medicine* 363: 2124–34.
4. Classen, D.C. et al. 2011. "'Global Trigger Tool' Shows That Adverse Events in Hospitals May Be Ten Times Greater Than Previously Measured." *Health Affairs* 30: 581–89.
5. Baker, G.R. et al. 2004. "The Canadian Adverse Events Study: The Incidence of Adverse Events among Hospital Patients in Canada." *Canadian Medical Association Journal* 170: 1678–86.
6. O'Hagan, J. et al. 2009. "Self-Reported Medical Errors in Seven Countries: Implications for Canada." *Healthcare Quarterly* 12: 55–61.
7. Charney, W. 2012. "Do No Harm?" *Canadian Dimension* 63, 3. May 10. Available at canadiandimension.com/articles/4671.
8. Wilson, R.M. et al. 1995. "The Quality in Australian Health Care Study." *Medical Journal of Australia* 163: 458–71.
9. Department of Health, United Kingdom. 2000. "An Organisation with a Memory. Report of an Expert Group on Learning from Adverse Events in the NHS." Chaired by the Chief Medical Officer. Available at dh.gov.uk/PublicationsAndStatistics.
10. Canadian Patient Safety Institute. 2012. "The Economics of Patient Safety in Acute Care." Available at patientsafetyinstitute.ca. Commissioned research.
11. Andel, C. et al. 2012. "The Economics of Health Care Quality and Medical Errors." *Journal of Health Care Finance* 39: 39–50.
12. Graedon, J. and T. Graedon. 2011. *Top Screwups Doctors Make and How to Avoid Them.* New York: Crown Archetype.

A Child Like Annie

1. Janvier, A. et al. 2012. "The Experience of Families with Children with Trisomy 13 and 18 in Social Networks." *Pediatrics* 130: 293–98.

A Doctor's Ordeal

1. In 1928 Sir Alexander Fleming observed that a type of penicillin mould could destroy colonies of *Staphylococcus aureus*. It was not until 1942, however, that a process for large-scale production of penicillin was developed by Howard Florey and Ernst Chain. Fleming, Florey and Chain shard the 1945 Nobel Prize in Medicine. Selman Waksman made the drug streptomycin from soil bacteria in 1943. Twelve years later, Lloyd Conover patented tetracycline, which became the most frequently prescribed broad-spectrum antibiotic in North America.

Special Recognition

1. 1996. "Cisapride: Arrhythmia Awareness." *Canadian Adverse Drug Reaction Newsletter* 6 (3):1–2.
2. Lee, P. 2001. "Deadly Prescription: Adverse Drug Reactions Kill an Estimated 10,000 Canadians Every Year." *Ottawa Citizen*, April 7.

Take Action

1. This letter was published on November 11, 2010, in the *Times and Transcript*, Moncton, New Brunswick. Reprinted with permission.

Not Too Late

1. Kellet, A.J. 1987. "Healing Angry Wounds: The Roles of Apology and Mediation in Disputes Between Physicians and Patients." *Missouri Journal of Dispute Resolution* 187: 111, citing R. Blum. 1960. *The Management of Doctor-Patient Relationship*. New York: McGraw-Hill.
2. Pelt, J.L. and L. Faldmo. 2008. "Physician Error and Disclosure." *Clinical Obstretrics and Gynecology* 51: 700–8.
3. Gomberg, F. "Apology for the Unexpected Death of a Child in a Healthcare Facility: A Prescription for Improvement." Available at www.riverdalemediation.com/resources/student-perspective-on-adr.

The Spark

1. Garros, D. et al. 2003. "Strangulation with Intravenous Tubing: A Previously Undescribed Adverse Event in Children." *Pediatrics* 111: 732–34.
2. Ibid.

Claire's Story

1. McGrath, R. 2009. "Claire's Story." *Canadian Nurse* 105: 28–30. Copyright Canadian Nurses Association. Reprinted with permission. Further reproduction prohibited.

Extraordinary People

1. Bernabé, C. and P. Daeninck. 2005. "Beauty Is Only Skin Deep: Prevalence of Dermatologic Disease in a Palliative Care Unit." *Journal of Pain and Symptom Management* 29: 419–22.

Whose Mistake?

1. Sibbald, R. et al. 2011. "A Checklist to Meet Ethical and Legal Obligations to Critically Ill Patients at the End of Life." *Healthcare Ethics* 14: 60–6.

Medical Malpractice

1. "Medical Malpractice" is adapted from: McKiggan, J.A. 2011. *Health Scare: The Consumer's Guide to Medical Malpractice Claims.* Available at apmlawyers.com.

FOR FURTHER INFORMATION

Selected Print Resources

Adamson, Catherine S. 2005. *Heidi Dawn Klompas: Missed Opportunities*. Vancouver: Catadam.

Banja, John. 2005. *Medical Errors and Medical Narcissism*. Boston: Jones and Bartlett.

Bannerman, Gary and Don Nixdorf. 2005. *Squandering Billions: Health Care in Canada*. Surrey: Hancock.

Berlinger, Nancy. 2005. *After Harm: Medical Error and the Ethics of Forgiveness*. Baltimore: John Hopkins University.

Charney, William, ed. 2012. *An Epidemic of Medical Errors and Hospital-Acquired Infections: Systemic and Social Causes*. Boca Raton: CRC.

Church, Rhonda and Neil MacKinnon. 2010. *Take as Directed: Your Prescription for Safe Health Care in Canada*. Toronto: ECW Press.

Cohen, Elizabeth. 2010. *The Empowered Patient: How to Get the Right Diagnosis, Buy the Cheapest Drugs, Beat Your Insurance Company, and Get the Best Medical Care Every Time*. New York: Ballantine.

Dekker, Sidney. 2011. *Patient Safety: A Human Factors Approach*. New York: CRC Press.

Ehrenchlou, Martine. 2012. *The Take-Charge Patient: How You Can Get the Best Medical Care*. Santa Monica: Lemon Grove.

Gawande, Atul. 2009. *The Checklist Manifesto: How to Get Things Right*. New York: Henry Holt.

Gibson, Rosemary and Janardan Prasad Singh. 2003. *Wall of Silence: The Untold Story of the Medical Mistakes That Kill and Injure Millions of Americans*. Washington, DC: LifeLine.

Gilbert, Sandra. 1997. *Wrongful Death: A Memoir.* New York: Norton.

Glouberman, Sholom. 2010. *My Operation: A Health Insider Becomes a Patient.* Toronto: Health and Everything.

Goldman, Brian. 2010. *The Night Shift.* Toronto: HarperCollins.

Groopman, Jerome. 2007. *How Doctors Think.* Boston: Houghton Mifflin.

Gupta, Sanjay. 2012. *Monday Mornings: A Novel.* New York: Grand Central.

Hallisy, Julia A. 2008. *The Empowered Patient: Hundreds of Life-Saving Facts, Action Steps and Strategies You Need to Know.* San Francisco: TheEmpoweredPatient.com.

Hicock, Larry with John Lewis. 2003. *Beware the Grieving Warrior: A Child's Preventable Death. A Struggle for Truth, Healing and Change.* Toronto: ECW Press.

Imber, Jonathan B. 2008. *Trusting Doctors: The Decline of Moral Authority in American Medicine.* Princeton: Princeton University.

Kenny, Charles. 2008. *The Best Practice: How the New Quality Movement Is Transforming Medicine.* New York: Public Affairs.

King, Sorrel. 2009. *Josie's Story: A Mother's Inspiring Crusade to Make Medical Care Safe.* New York: Atlantic.

Makary, Marty. 2012. *Unaccountable: What Hospitals Won't Tell You and How Transparency Can Revolutionize Health Care.* New York: Bloomsbury.

McIver, Susan B. 2001. *Medical Nightmares: The Human Face of Errors.* Toronto: Chestnut.

Moynihan, Ray and Alan Cassels. 2006. *Selling Sickness: How the World's Biggest Pharmaceutical Companies Are Turning Us All into Patients.* Vancouver: Greystone.

Null, Gary et al. 2010. *Death by Medicine.* Mount Jackson: Praktikos.

Pronovost, Peter and Eric Vohr. 2010. *Safe Patients, Smart Hospitals: How One Doctor's Checklist Can Help Us Change Health Care from the Inside Out.* New York: Hudson Street.

Richardson, William C., Chair, Committee on Quality Health Care in America. 2001. *Crossing the Quality Chasm: A New Health Care System for the 21st Century.* Washington, DC: National Academy.

Salas, Eduardo and Karen Frush. 2012. *Improving Patient Safety through Teamwork and Team Training.* Oxford: Oxford University.

Simpson, Jeffrey. 2012. *Chronic Condition.* Toronto: Allen Lane.

Sloan, John. 2009. *A Bitter Pill: How the Medical System Is Failing the Elderly.* Vancouver: Greystone.

Truog, Robert, David M. Browning and Judith A. Johnson. 2011. *Talking with Patients and Families about Medical Error: A Guide for Education and Practice.* Baltimore: John Hopkins University.

Wachter, Robert. 2012. *Understanding Patient Safety* 2nd ed. New York: McGraw Medical.

Wachter, Robert M. and Kaveh G. Shojania. 2004. *Internal Bleeding: The Truth Behind America's Terrifying Epidemic of Medical Mistakes.* New York: Rugged Land.

Wojcieszak, Douglas. 2013. *Did the Doctor Make a Mistake? A Guide for Patients and Families Facing Complications and Possible Medical Errors.* Glen Carbon, Illinois: Sorry Works.

Young, Terence H. 2009. *Death by Prescription: A Father Takes on His Daughter's Killer: The Multi-Billion-Dollar Pharmaceutical Industry.* Toronto: Key Porter.

Youngberg, Barbara J. 2012. *Patient Safety Handbook.* Boston: Jones and Bartlett.

Selected Electronic Resources

World Health Organization
World Alliance for Patient Safety: who.int/patientsafety/worldalliance/en/
Patients for Patient Safety: who.int/patientsafety/patients_for_patient/en/

Australia
Australian Commission on Safety and Quality in Health Care: aihw.gov.au
Australian Patient Safety Foundation: www.apsf.net.au

Canada
Canadian Institute for Health Information: cihi.ca
Canadian Institute for Health Research: cihr.ca
Canadian Patient Safety Institute: patientsafetyinstitute.ca

Institute for Safe Medication Practices in Canada: ismp-canada.org
Manitoba Institute for Patient Safety: mbips.ca
Patients' Association of Canada: patientsassociation.ca
Patients for Patient Safety Canada: patientsforpatientsafety.ca
Safer Health Care Now!: saferhealthcarenow.ca

Denmark
Danish Society for Patient Safety: patientsikkerhed.dk/en

Europe
European Network for Patient Safety and Quality of Health Care: eu-patient.eu

Germany
German Agency for Quality in Medicine: aqumed.de
German Coalition for Patient Safety: german-coalition-for-patient-safety.org

Israel
Israel Center for Medical Simulation: msr.org.il

New Zealand
New Zealand Health Quality and Safety Commission: hqsc.govt.nz

United Kingdom
Clinical Human Factors Group: chfg.org
Health Foundation: health.org.uk
National Institute for Health and Clinical Excellence: nice.org.uk
National Patient Safety Agency: npsa.nhs.uk

United States
Agency for Healthcare Research and Quality: ahrq.gov
Anesthesia Patient Safety Foundation: apsf.org
Empowered Patient: theempoweredpatient.com
Empowered Patient Coalition: empoweredpatientcoalition.org
Institute for Healthcare Improvement: ihi.org
Institute for Patient and Family Centered Care: ipfcc.org
Institute for Safe Medication Practices: ismp.org
Joint Commission: jointcommission.org
Josie King Foundation: josieking.org
Leap Frog: leapfroggroup.org
Medically Induced Trauma Support Services: mitss.org

Mothers Against Medical Error: mamemomsonline.org
National Center for Patient Safety: www.patientsafety.gov
National Patient Safety Foundation: npsf.org
National Quality Forum: qualityforum.org
PULSE (Persons United Limiting Substandards and Errors in Health Care): pulseamerica.org
Safe Care Campaign: safecarecampaign.org

SUSAN MCIVER holds a Ph.D. in entomology/microbiology, was a professor at the University of Toronto with appointments to the Faculty of Medicine and a department chair at the University of Guelph. Subsequently, she served as a community coroner in British Columbia. She is also the author of *Medical Nightmares: The Human Face of Errors*.

ROBIN WYNDHAM was a registered nurse for 34 years. She worked in neonatal intensive care, surgery, psychiatry and residential care and had a special interest in palliative care. She studied nursing at the Vancouver General Hospital and English at the University of British Columbia.

DISCARD

GET *the* eBOOK FREE

PROOF OF
PURCHASE
REQUIRED

At ECW Press, we want you to enjoy this book in what-ever format you like, whenever you like. Leave your print book at home and take the eBook to go! Purchase the print edition and receive the eBook free. Just send an email to ebook@ecwpress.com and include:

- the book title
- the name of the store where you purchased it
- your receipt number
- your preference of file type: PDF or ePub?

A real person will respond to your email with your eBook attached. And thanks for supporting an independently owned Canadian publisher with your purchase!